PILATES BAR WORKOUT

Raise the Bar on Your Fitness, Get Fit and Fabulous with this Dynamic Pilates Approach to Sculpting a Stronger, Leaner You

Norman W. Greenberg

CONTENTS

INTRODUCTION

Welcome to the world of Pilates Bar Workout, where total-body transformation is within reach.

I have always been passionate about fitness and wellness. Over the years, I have tried many different workout routines, but it wasn't until I discovered Pilates bar workout that I truly found my calling.

I decided to write this book because I wanted to share my knowledge and experience with others who are interested in Pilates bar workout or who are looking for a new way to stay fit and healthy. I understand that embarking on a new workout routine can be overwhelming, and there is a lot of information available that can be confusing and contradictory. Through this book, I aim to provide you with a clear understanding of Pilates Bar Workout, its benefits, and how to incorporate it into your fitness routine.

Pilates Bar Workout is a versatile exercise regimen that can benefit people of all ages and fitness levels. Its emphasis on controlled movements, core strengthening, and flexibility can help improve posture, balance, and overall fitness.

In these pages, you will find detailed explanations and step-by-step instructions for a wide range of Pilates bar workout exercises and also gain practical knowledge on how to perform each exercise correctly, avoiding any potential injuries or setbacks. You will also gain insight into the different variations of Pilates Bar Workout, including those designed for weight loss, injury prevention, stress relief, and athletic training.

I wrote this book with the belief that everyone can benefit from Pilates bar workout, regardless of their current fitness level or experience. I hope that this book will serve as a valuable resource for anyone looking to improve their health and wellbeing, and that it will inspire you to embark on your own Pilates bar workout journey.

I'm excited to share my knowledge and expertise with you, and to help you achieve your fitness and wellness goals through Pilates Bar Workout. Let's get started on this journey together.

CHAPTER 1: THE FUNDAMENTALS OF PILATES BAR WORKOUTS

What is a Pilates Bar and What is Pilates Bar Workout?

Pilates is a low-impact exercise regimen that focuses on developing strength, flexibility, and endurance in the body's core muscles. It was developed by Joseph Pilates in the early 20th century, and since then, it has become increasingly popular due to its numerous health benefits. Pilates Bar workout is a variation of Pilates that utilizes a long, lightweight bar to perform exercises that enhance the strength and flexibility of the body.

The Pilates Bar, also known as the Pilates Stick or Pilates Rod, Is a lightweight and flexible bar that ranges in length from four to six feet. It is typically made of aluminum or other lightweight materials and has adjustable resistance bands that attach to either end of the bar. The bar is designed to provide resistance to your movements, making your exercises more challenging and effective.

Pilates Bar workouts use the Pilates Bar to provide resistance and support during exercises, which helps to build core strength, improve balance and stability, and increase flexibility. The Pilates Bar is also used to help align the body properly during exercises, which can help to prevent injuries and promote proper form.

Pilates Bar workouts typically involve a series of controlled movements that focus on specific muscle groups. These movements are designed to improve strength, flexibility, and balance. Pilates Bar workouts can be done alone or in a group setting, and they can be tailored to suit the needs and fitness levels of individuals of all ages and fitness levels.

There are many different types of Pilates Bar workouts, and each one is designed to target specific muscle groups and improve overall fitness. Some of the most popular Pilates Bar workouts include the Pilates Roll-Up, the Pilates Teaser, the Pilates Double Leg Stretch, and the Pilates Plank. Each of these exercises uses the Pilates Bar to provide resistance and support, which helps to build strength and improve flexibility.

How Does a Pilates Bar Work

So, how does a Pilates bar work? The concept is simple: the bar serves as a prop that provides resistance to your muscles as you perform various exercises. The resistance helps to engage and challenge your muscles, leading to increased strength and toning. The bar also provides stability, allowing you to perform movements with greater control and precision.

The design of the Pilates bar is straightforward. It consists of a long, lightweight metal or wooden bar with adjustable resistance bands on either end. The resistance bands are made of high-quality elastic and come in varying strengths, allowing you to adjust the resistance to match your fitness level and the specific exercises you are performing.

To use the Pilates bar, you simply hold onto the resistance bands and perform a series of exercises that target your upper and lower body, core, and back muscles. The exercises are often performed while standing, sitting, or lying on a mat, and range from simple movements to more advanced, challenging exercises that require greater strength, balance, and coordination.

Some of the most common exercises performed with the Pilates bar include squats, lunges, bicep curls, tricep extensions, and chest presses. These exercises target specific muscle groups in your body, helping to improve muscle tone, strength, and flexibility. By using the Pilates bar, you can also perform exercises that are difficult or impossible to do with traditional strength-training equipment, such as dumbbells or resistance bands.

The Benefits of Pilates Bar Workout: What You Need to Know

While many people are familiar with traditional Pilates exercises, the addition of a bar to the workout offers a whole new set of benefits that are worth exploring.

Pilates bar workout allows you to target multiple muscle groups at once. By incorporating resistance from the bar, you can engage more muscles with each movement, resulting in a more effective workout. This can help you build strength and tone your entire body, while also improving your balance and stability.

Another benefit of Pilates bar workout is that it is low-impact and gentle on the joints. Unlike high-intensity workouts that can be hard on your body, Pilates bar workout focuses on controlled movements and proper alignment. This means that you can get a challenging workout without putting unnecessary strain on your joints.

One key benefit of Pilates bar workout is its ability to improve overall body strength. By incorporating the use of a bar, this workout provides additional resistance and challenge that can help build muscle and increase stamina. This makes it an ideal workout for athletes and anyone looking to build overall strength and endurance.

Another major benefit of Pilates bar workout is its ability to improve flexibility and mobility. The workout focuses on controlled, precise movements that stretch and strengthen the body, leading to increased range of motion and improved joint health. This can be particularly beneficial for older adults or those with joint pain or mobility issues.

Pilates bar workout is also a highly effective way to improve posture and balance. The workout targets the core muscles that support the spine and promotes proper alignment, which can lead to improved posture and balance over time. This can be particularly beneficial for people who spend long hours sitting at a desk or for anyone looking to improve their overall posture.

Finally, Pilates bar workout offers a unique mind-body connection that can help reduce stress and improve overall well-being. By focusing on controlled movements and breath work, this workout can help promote relaxation and mindfulness, which can have a positive impact on both physical and mental health.

The Fundamentals of Pilates: Understanding the Basics

In this section, we will delve into the fundamentals of Pilates, exploring the basic principles and techniques that underpin this dynamic exercise system. By understanding these fundamentals, you can gain a deeper appreciation for Pilates and its many benefits.

Breathing

One of the key principles of Pilates is breath control. Proper breathing is essential to performing Pilates exercises correctly, as it helps to regulate the movement of the body and promote relaxation. In Pilates, breath control is achieved through diaphragmatic breathing, which involves inhaling deeply through the nose and exhaling slowly through the mouth. This breathing technique helps to engage the core muscles and promote relaxation, which is essential to performing Pilates exercises effectively.

Alignment

Another important aspect of Pilates is alignment. Proper alignment is essential to ensure that the body is properly supported during each exercise. In Pilates, proper alignment involves maintaining a neutral spine, with the shoulders relaxed and the pelvis properly aligned. By maintaining proper alignment, the body is better able to engage the correct muscles and avoid injury.

Centering

Pilates also emphasizes the importance of centering, which involves engaging the core muscles to support the spine and promote proper alignment. The core muscles include the muscles of the abdomen, lower back, and hips, and are essential to performing Pilates exercises effectively. By focusing on centering, Pilates helps to promote a strong, stable core, which is essential to overall health and fitness.

Control

Another key principle of Pilates is control. Pilates exercises are designed to be performed slowly and with precision, allowing for maximum control over the movement of the body. By performing exercises slowly and with control, the body is better able to engage the correct muscles and avoid injury. Control is also essential to achieving the maximum benefit from each exercise.

Precision

Precision is another important principle of Pilates. Pilates exercises are designed to be performed with a high degree of precision, with each movement performed with care and attention to detail. By focusing on precision, Pilates helps to promote proper alignment and engage the correct muscles, leading to better results and a reduced risk of injury.

Flow

Finally, Pilates emphasizes the importance of flow. Pilates exercises are designed to be performed in a flowing, continuous manner, with each movement seamlessly transitioning into the next. By performing exercises in a flowing manner, the body is better able to engage the correct muscles and achieve maximum benefit from each exercise.

By mastering these basic principles, you can improve their form, technique, and overall effectiveness of their workout.

CHAPTER 2: SETTING UP YOUR PILATES BAR WORKOUT

The Importance of Proper Alignment and Posture

In the world of fitness, there are few things more important than proper alignment and posture. These elements not only help to prevent injury but also improve the effectiveness of your workout. This is particularly true when it comes to Pilates, where proper alignment and posture are essential for maximizing the benefits of your workout.

So, why is alignment so important in Pilates? First and foremost, it helps you engage the right muscles during each exercise. When your body is properly aligned, your muscles are able to work together more efficiently, which can help you achieve better results in less time. Additionally, proper alignment can help prevent injury by reducing strain on your joints and other sensitive areas of the body.

But what does proper alignment actually look like in Pilates? It starts with the feet. Your feet should be hip-distance apart and parallel, with your weight evenly distributed between them. From there, your knees should be slightly bent, and your pelvis should be in a neutral position, with your lower back gently pressing into the mat. Moving up the body, your shoulders should be relaxed and down, away from your ears, and your arms should be long and extended. Your neck should be in a neutral position, with your gaze focused straight ahead.

Of course, achieving proper alignment is easier said than done. It requires a lot of practice and a deep understanding of your body's mechanics. That's why it's so important to work with a trained Pilates instructor who can guide you through the process and help you make the most of each exercise.

Beyond proper alignment, good posture is also essential for a successful Pilates practice. When you have good posture, your body is in a state of balance, with each part working together to support the whole. This not only helps you avoid injury but also allows you to move with greater ease and grace.

To achieve good posture in Pilates, start by focusing on the three natural curves of the spine: the cervical, thoracic, and lumbar curves. These curves should be present and properly aligned during each exercise, with the head, neck, and shoulders stacked above the pelvis and the lower back gently pressing into the mat.

As you move through each exercise, pay close attention to your body and make adjustments as needed. Remember, proper alignment and posture are not something you achieve once and forget about; they require constant attention and refinement.

Choosing the Right Equipment for Your Workout

When it comes to Pilates bar workouts, selecting the right equipment is crucial for a safe and effective workout. In this section, we will discuss the different types of equipment available and how to choose the right one for your needs.

One of the most important pieces of equipment in Pilates bar workouts is the bar itself. There are various types of bars available, including wooden, metal, and plastic. Wooden bars are typically preferred for their durability and grip, while metal and plastic bars are more affordable and lightweight.

Another essential piece of equipment is the mat. Mats provide cushioning and support for the body during exercises, helping to reduce the risk of injury. When choosing a mat, consider factors such as thickness, texture, and size.

In addition to the bar and mat, there are also various accessories that can enhance your Pilates bar workout. These include resistance bands, balls, and weights. Resistance bands are particularly useful for adding resistance to exercises, while balls and weights can be used to target specific muscle groups.

When selecting equipment for your Pilates bar workout, it is important to consider your fitness level and personal preferences. If you are just starting out, a basic set of equipment may be all you need. As you progress, you may want to invest in additional equipment to challenge yourself and take your workouts to the next level.

It is also essential to choose high-quality equipment that is safe and reliable. Look for equipment that has been tested and certified by reputable organizations, and be sure to read reviews and check the manufacturer's warranty before making a purchase.

Pre-Workout Preparation: Stretching and Warm-Up Exercises

Pre-workout preparation is a crucial component of any exercise routine, including Pilates bar workouts. In this section, we will discuss the importance of stretching and warm-up exercises and how to incorporate them into your Pilates bar workout.

Stretching is an essential part of any workout routine as it helps to increase flexibility, prevent injury, and improve overall performance. Before starting your Pilates bar workout, take a few minutes to perform a series of dynamic stretches that focus on the muscles you will be using during your workout.

Dynamic stretching involves moving through a range of motion, rather than holding a static stretch. This type of stretching is particularly effective for preparing the body for exercise and can help to increase blood flow and warm up the muscles.

Some effective dynamic stretching exercises for Pilates bar workouts include:

Arm Swings

This exercise primarily targets the shoulders, chest, and upper back, and can help to increase range of motion, flexibility, and blood flow to the upper body.

To perform arm swings, start by standing tall with your feet hip-width apart and your arms extended straight out to the sides at shoulder height. Your palms should be facing forward. Begin swinging your arms forward and backward, gradually increasing the range of motion until your arms are swinging in large circles. Keep your core engaged and your spine straight throughout the movement. You can also vary the direction of the swings by rotating your arms inwards or outwards.

It's Important to keep the movements smooth and controlled, and to avoid any jerky or sudden movements that could lead to injury. You should also be aware of your breathing, inhaling as you swing your arms forward and exhaling as you swing them back.

Hip Circles

This target the hip muscles and help to improve flexibility and mobility in the hip joint. To perform this exercise, stand with your feet hip-width apart, and place your hands on your hips. Slowly start to circle your hips in a clockwise direction, making small circles at first, then gradually increasing the size of the circles. Make sure to keep your feet flat on the ground and your torso still, and focus on moving your hips smoothly and evenly.

After a few rotations, switch to counterclockwise circles, again starting with small circles and gradually increasing the size. Remember to keep your movements slow and controlled, and try to maintain a steady pace throughout the exercise. You can also vary the speed and size of the circles as you become more comfortable with the movement.

Hip circles can help to release tension and stiffness in the hip joints, which can be especially beneficial for people who spend a lot of time sitting or standing in one position. This exercise can also help to improve balance and stability by engaging the core muscles and promoting proper alignment in the lower body.

If you have any pre-existing hip conditions or injuries, it's always a good idea to check with a healthcare provider or qualified fitness professional before trying this or any new exercise.

Leg Swings

To perform leg swings, begin by standing with your feet hip-width apart and holding onto the Pilates bar for support. Keep your core engaged and maintain good posture throughout the exercise. Then, swing one leg forward and backward, keeping it straight and raising it as high as is comfortable for you. Repeat this motion for 10-15 repetitions on each leg, gradually increasing the height of your swing.

Next, swing your leg side-to-side in a sweeping motion, again keeping it straight and controlled. Repeat for 10-15 repetitions on each leg.

When performing leg swings, be mindful not to swing too forcefully or jerk the leg. Focus on controlled, fluid movements that engage the muscles of the hip and leg. Also, be sure to maintain good balance and control throughout the exercise to avoid injury.

The Cat-Cow Stretch

The cat-cow stretch is a great way to warm up your spine.

To perform the cat-cow stretch, start on your hands and knees with your wrists directly under your shoulders and your knees under your hips. Begin by inhaling and arching your spine, allowing your belly to drop towards the floor and your head to lift towards the ceiling. This is the cow portion of the stretch. Then, as you exhale, round your spine towards the ceiling and tuck your chin towards your chest. This is the cat portion of the stretch. Repeat this movement, inhaling as you arch and exhaling as you round, for several repetitions.

It's Important to move smoothly and slowly through the cat-cow stretch, focusing on your breath and maintaining control throughout the movement. Avoid forcing your range of motion and be mindful of any discomfort or pain in your back or neck. This exercise is great for beginners, but can also be modified to make it more challenging by adding arm or leg movements.

Shoulder Rolls

Shoulder rolls help to improve the flexibility and mobility of your shoulders.

To perform shoulder rolls, stand up straight with your feet shoulder-width apart and your arms at your sides. Slowly raise your shoulders towards your ears, hold for a few seconds, and then roll your shoulders back and down. Repeat this movement for several repetitions, aiming to create a circular motion with your shoulders.

As you perform shoulder rolls, it is important to keep your neck relaxed and to breathe deeply and evenly. You should also be aware of any tension or discomfort in your shoulders and neck, and adjust the intensity of the exercise accordingly.

In addition to improving shoulder mobility, shoulder rolls can also help to increase blood flow to the upper body and reduce tension and stress in the shoulders and neck. When incorporating shoulder rolls into your warm-up routine, aim to perform them for at least 30 seconds to one minute, gradually increasing the number of repetitions or the duration of the exercise as your shoulder mobility improves.

The Lunge with a Twist

This exercise targets the lower body, specifically the quadriceps, hamstrings, and glutes, while also engaging the core and promoting flexibility in the thoracic spine.

To perform the lunge with a twist, begin in a standing position with your feet hip-width apart. Step one foot forward, keeping your knee directly over your ankle, and lower your back knee towards the ground, creating a 90-degree angle in both legs. Keep your torso upright and engage your core to stabilize your body.

Once you are in the lunge position, rotate your torso towards your front knee, twisting your spine and placing your opposite elbow on the inside of your front knee. Hold this position for a few seconds before rotating back to center and returning to a standing position. Repeat on the other side, stepping the opposite foot forward into the lunge and twisting towards that knee.

It is important to maintain proper form throughout the exercise. Keep your front knee directly over your ankle, and avoid letting it collapse inward or outward. Engage your core muscles to stabilize your torso and prevent any twisting in your lower back. Additionally, make sure to perform the exercise in a slow and controlled manner, avoiding any sudden or jerky movements.

Side Bends

Side bends are a great stretching and warm-up exercise for Pilates bar workout that target the obliques, back, and hips. Here's how to perform the exercise:

1. Begin by standing with your feet hip-distance apart and holding onto the Pilates bar with both hands. Your arms should be extended overhead, with the bar resting on your shoulders.
2. Inhale and reach your arms up towards the ceiling, lengthening your spine and engaging your core.
3. Exhale and slowly lean to the right, keeping your shoulders level and your hips facing forward. Allow your left arm to reach up and over your head, stretching your left side.
4. Inhale and return to the starting position, then exhale and repeat on the other side.
5. Repeat the exercise for 8-10 repetitions on each side.

When performing side bends, it's important to keep your core engaged and your shoulders relaxed. Avoid letting your hips tilt to one side, and instead keep them facing forward to maintain proper alignment.

Knee Lift

Knee Lifts are a type of warm-up exercise that target the abdominal muscles, hip flexors, and lower back. This exercise is often performed using the Pilates Bar, which is a long metal or wooden bar with attached resistance bands that provide tension to the muscles during movement.

To perform Knee Lifts with the Pilates Bar, follow these steps:

1. Start by lying down on your back with your knees bent and your feet flat on the ground. Hold the Pilates Bar with both hands and place it on top of your shins, just below your knees.
2. Engage your abdominal muscles by drawing your navel in towards your spine. This will help stabilize your pelvis and protect your lower back.
3. Slowly lift your feet off the ground, keeping your knees bent at a 90-degree angle. As you do this, lift the Pilates Bar off your shins and bring it towards your chest.
4. Hold this position for a few seconds, then slowly lower your feet and the Pilates Bar back to the starting position.
5. Repeat this movement for several repetitions, focusing on maintaining control and stability throughout the exercise.

When performing Knee Lifts with the Pilates Bar, it's important to maintain proper form to prevent injury and get the most benefit from the exercise. Here are some tips to keep in mind:

- Keep your feet together and your knees in line with your hips throughout the exercise.
- Avoid lifting your shoulders off the ground, as this can strain your neck and upper back.
- Breathe deeply and exhale as you lift your feet and the Pilates Bar towards your chest.

- Use the resistance of the Pilates Bar to engage your abdominal muscles and deepen the stretch in your hip flexors.

Torso Twists

This exercise focuses on the core muscles of your body, including your abs and obliques.

To perform this exercise, start by sitting on the floor with your legs crossed in front of you. Place your left hand on your right knee and your right hand behind you on the floor. Inhale deeply and lengthen your spine, sitting up tall. As you exhale, gently twist your torso to the right, using your left hand to deepen the stretch. Hold the stretch for a few seconds, then inhale as you return to center. Repeat on the other side, placing your right hand on your left knee and your left hand behind you on the floor.

It's important to keep your spine straight and tall throughout the exercise, avoiding slouching or rounding your shoulders. You can deepen the stretch by using your hand to gently guide your knee further towards the floor. However, be careful not to push yourself too far and cause any pain or discomfort.

Pelvic Tilts

Pelvic tilts help to warm up and activate the muscles in your lower back, abdominals, and pelvic area. This exercise involves gently tilting your pelvis forward and backward in a controlled motion, which helps to improve flexibility, stability, and alignment of your spine.

Here's how to perform pelvic tilts:

1. Lie down on your back with your knees bent and your feet flat on the floor.
2. Place your arms by your sides, palms down.
3. Inhale and tilt your pelvis forward, allowing your lower back to arch slightly.
4. Exhale and tilt your pelvis backward, flattening your lower back against the floor.
5. Repeat for several reps, moving slowly and smoothly.

As you perform pelvic tilts, pay attention to the movement in your lower back and pelvis. You should feel a gentle stretch in your lower back as you tilt your pelvis forward, and a contraction in your abdominals as you tilt your pelvis backward. It's important to perform pelvic tilts in a slow and controlled manner, and avoid arching your back too much or forcing the movement.

CHAPTER 3: THE FOUNDATION OF PILATES BAR WORKOUT

The Art of Breathing: How to Breathe for Optimal Results

The art of breathing is an integral part of Pilates bar workout. Proper breathing techniques can improve the effectiveness of your workout, as well as your overall health and well-being. Breathing is an essential component of Pilates exercises, and it helps to engage the right muscles and maintain proper alignment.

When you inhale, the muscles in your body expand, and when you exhale, they contract. This process is crucial in Pilates bar workout, where the emphasis is on controlled movements and correct posture. Proper breathing can also help to reduce stress, improve circulation, and increase your overall endurance.

To breathe correctly during Pilates bar workout, you need to focus on breathing from your diaphragm. This means inhaling deeply through your nose, filling your lungs completely, and then exhaling through your mouth, slowly and steadily. It's important to breathe deeply and consistently throughout each exercise, and to avoid holding your breath or taking shallow breaths.

In Pilates bar workout, there are specific breathing patterns that are designed to enhance the benefits of each exercise. For example, during certain exercises, you may be instructed to inhale deeply as you prepare for the movement, and then exhale as you perform it.

Other exercises may require you to hold your breath for a brief moment at the top of the movement before exhaling.

Some essential breathing techniques are:

Diaphragmatic Breathing

Diaphragmatic breathing is a breathing technique that emphasizes the use of the diaphragm to breathe more deeply and efficiently.

To perform diaphragmatic breathing, start by sitting or lying down in a comfortable position. Place one hand on your chest and the other on your abdomen, just below your ribcage. Take a slow, deep breath in through your nose, filling your lungs with air and allowing your abdomen to expand. As you exhale through your mouth, imagine that you are drawing your navel towards your spine and feel your abdomen contract. Continue breathing in this manner, focusing on the rise and fall of your abdomen rather than your chest.

It's Important to note that diaphragmatic breathing should not feel forced or uncomfortable. If you feel lightheaded or dizzy, take a break and return to normal breathing. With practice, you will become more comfortable with this technique and it will become a natural part of your breathing pattern.

In Pilates bar workout, diaphragmatic breathing is often used during exercises that require core stability and control, such as planks and leg lifts. By focusing on your breath, you can maintain proper form and alignment, which helps to prevent injury and maximize the benefits of the exercise.

Thoracic Breathing

Thoracic breathing facilitate deep breathing and optimize oxygenation of the body. This type of breathing involves expanding the rib cage and the upper chest area rather than the belly, as in diaphragmatic breathing. Thoracic breathing helps to activate the muscles of the upper body and improve posture.

To practice thoracic breathing, begin by sitting or standing tall with your shoulders relaxed. Inhale deeply through your nose, focusing on expanding your ribcage outward and upward, filling your lungs from the top down. Your shoulders should remain relaxed and stationary, while your upper chest expands. Then, exhale through your mouth, gently contracting your abdominal muscles to help expel the air from your lungs.

It's Important to remember to keep your breaths slow and controlled, and to avoid lifting your shoulders or tensing your neck while inhaling. Thoracic breathing can also be done while performing Pilates Bar exercises, such as the plank or the bridge, to enhance their benefits. Regular practice of thoracic breathing can help to increase lung capacity, reduce stress and anxiety, and improve overall posture and alignment.

Ribcage Breathing

Ribcage breathing is a breathing technique that emphasizes expanding the ribcage during inhalation and contracting it during exhalation.

To perform ribcage breathing, start by sitting or standing tall with your shoulders relaxed and your spine in a neutral position. Place your hands on your ribcage, with your fingertips resting on the sides of your body and your thumbs in the back. Inhale deeply through your nose, expanding your ribcage out to the sides and back, but keeping your belly button drawn towards your spine. As you exhale through your mouth, imagine gently pulling your ribcage inwards towards your center and feeling your deep core muscles engage.

Repeat this sequence for a few breaths, focusing on the expansion and contraction of your ribcage with each inhale and exhale.

Lateral Breathing

Lateral breathing is a fundamental breathing technique that involves breathing deeply into the lower part of the lungs, while expanding the ribcage laterally.

To practice lateral breathing, start by finding a comfortable seated or lying down position. Place your hands on the sides of your ribcage, with your thumbs pointing towards your back. Inhale deeply, feeling the expansion of your ribcage laterally, and exhale slowly, feeling the contraction of your ribcage towards the center of your body.

As you practice lateral breathing, focus on keeping your chest and shoulders relaxed, and let the movement of your ribcage be the main driver of the breath. Try to avoid shallow breathing or letting your chest rise and fall with each breath, as this can limit the amount of oxygen that reaches your muscles and prevent you from achieving optimal results.

The 3-part Breath

The 3-part breath is a powerful breathing technique used in Pilates bar workouts to help practitioners gain control of their breath and bring their focus inward. This technique involves inhaling deeply, first into the belly, then into the lower chest, and finally into the upper chest.

To practice the 3-part breath, start by finding a comfortable seated or lying position. Close your eyes and bring your attention to your breath. Take a deep inhale through your nose and allow your belly to expand fully. Then, continue the inhale and bring the breath into your lower chest, feeling your ribs expand. Finally, complete the inhale and bring the breath into your upper chest, feeling your chest expand fully.

Hold the breath for a few seconds, and then exhale slowly and completely through your mouth, releasing the air from your upper chest, lower chest, and belly in sequence. Repeat this cycle for several breaths, focusing on the sensation of the breath moving through your body and the relaxation it brings.

Breath Retention

Breath retention is a powerful breathing technique used in Pilates Bar workout that involves inhaling deeply, retaining the breath for a few seconds, and then exhaling slowly. This technique is also known as Kumbhaka or "breath holding" in yoga.

To perform breath retention, begin by taking a slow, deep breath in through your nose, filling your lungs completely. Hold your breath for a few seconds before slowly exhaling through your mouth. As you exhale, try to release any tension in your body and feel your muscles relaxing.

Breath retention helps to increase lung capacity and improve oxygenation of the blood, which can lead to improved performance during your Pilates Bar workout. Additionally, holding your breath can activate the parasympathetic nervous system, which promotes relaxation and reduces stress.

It is important to practice breath retention under the guidance of a certified Pilates instructor or yoga teacher, as it can be challenging and potentially dangerous if done incorrectly. Beginners should start with short breath holds and gradually work up to longer periods of retention as they become more comfortable with the technique.

The Sighing Breath

The "Sighing Breath" technique is a deep and relaxing breath that can help to release tension and promote a sense of calm during your Pilates Bar workout. This technique involves taking a long, slow inhale through the nose, and then exhaling through the mouth with a soft, audible sigh.

To perform this technique, find a comfortable seated or lying position with your spine in a neutral position. Take a deep inhale through your nose, filling your lungs with air. Then, exhale slowly through your mouth with a gentle sigh, letting the breath flow out smoothly and evenly.

As you exhale, focus on releasing any tension or stress in your body. Imagine that you are letting go of any negative energy or emotions with each exhale, and feel your body becoming more relaxed and at ease with each breath.

You can practice the Sighing Breath technique at any time during your Pilates Bar workout, but it is especially beneficial during the warm-up and cool-down periods. It can also be helpful to use this technique if you feel tense or stressed during the workout, or if you need a moment to refocus and center yourself.

The Counted Breath

The Counted Breath is a breathing technique used to help practitioners synchronize their breath with their movements. This technique helps to improve focus and concentration during exercises and can lead to better results.

To practice the Counted Breath, start by standing with your feet shoulder-width apart and your hands resting on your hips. Inhale deeply through your nose, filling your lungs with air. As you exhale, count to five and contract your abdominal muscles, pulling your navel towards your spine. Hold your breath for a count of two, and then inhale again for a count of five, expanding your ribcage and lifting your chest. Repeat this pattern for several breaths, gradually increasing the length of your inhale and exhale counts.

As you practice the Counted Breath, focus on keeping your breath slow and steady, and try to maintain a consistent rhythm. This technique can be used during a variety of Pilates Bar exercises, including squats, lunges, and leg lifts.

Ocean Breath

Ocean Breath is a type of breathing technique used in Pilates Bar workouts to increase mindfulness, reduce stress, and promote relaxation. It is also known as Ujjayi breath, which is a Sanskrit word meaning "victorious breath."

To practice Ocean Breath, start by sitting in a comfortable position with your back straight and your eyes closed. Take a deep inhale through your nose, filling your lungs with air. As you exhale through your nose, constrict the back of your throat to create a "hissing" sound in the back of your throat.

Imagine that you are fogging up a mirror with your breath. You should feel the air passing through your nostrils and into the back of your throat. Your breath should be slow, deep, and controlled.

Practice Ocean Breath for a few minutes at the beginning of your Pilates Bar workout, and then continue to use it throughout your workout to help you stay focused and centered. As you become more comfortable with this technique, you can increase the length of your inhales and exhales.

Alternate Nostril Breathing

Alternate Nostril Breathing is a breathing technique used in Pilates bar workout that helps to promote calmness and relaxation while also improving focus and concentration. This technique involves the use of the fingers to alternately block one nostril while inhaling and exhaling through the other.

To practice this technique, begin by sitting comfortably with a straight spine and relaxed shoulders. Use the right hand to bring the index and middle fingers to rest on the space between the eyebrows, with the thumb resting on the right nostril and the ring finger on the left nostril.

Start by blocking the right nostril with your thumb and inhale deeply through the left nostril. At the end of the inhale, close off the left nostril with your ring finger and hold the breath briefly. Next, release the right nostril and exhale fully through it. At the end of the exhale, inhale deeply through the right nostril, close it off with the thumb, and hold the breath briefly. Finally, release the left nostril and exhale fully through it. This completes one round of alternate nostril breathing.

It's important to remember to breathe slowly and deeply throughout the practice, without straining or forcing the breath. Start with a few rounds of alternate nostril breathing and gradually work your way up to longer sessions as your comfort level and familiarity with the technique increases.

Connecting Mind and Body: Focusing on Your Mind-Body Connection

When it comes to Pilates bar workout, it's not just about the physical movements. One of the core principles of Pilates is to connect the mind and body to achieve optimal results. This connection, also known as the mind-body connection, involves focusing on the present moment and being mindful of the movements you're performing.

The mind-body connection is an important aspect of Pilates, and it starts with your breath. Breathing is a fundamental part of Pilates, and it can help you to connect your mind and body. As you breathe, you can focus your attention on your movements, which can help you to move more efficiently and effectively. Breathing can also help you to relax and calm your mind, which can help you to achieve better results.

In addition to breathing, there are other techniques that can help you to connect your mind and body during your Pilates bar workout. These include visualization, concentration, and mindfulness. Visualization involves picturing yourself performing the movement correctly in your mind's eye before actually performing it. Concentration involves focusing your attention on the specific muscles you are using during the movement. Mindfulness involves being aware of the present moment and fully engaging in the movement.

To connect your mind and body during your Pilates bar workout, it is important to be present in the moment. This means paying attention to your body and your movements, rather than allowing your mind to wander. By being present, you can improve your focus and concentration, which can help you to achieve better results.

One technique that can help you to connect your mind and body during your Pilates bar workout is visualization. Visualization involves picturing yourself performing the movement correctly in your mind's eye before actually performing it. This can help you to improve your form and technique, which can lead to better results. Visualization can also help you to stay focused and motivated during your workout.

Another technique that can help you to connect your mind and body during your Pilates bar workout is concentration. Concentration involves focusing your attention on the specific muscles you are using during the movement. By focusing your attention, you can improve your form and technique, which can lead to better results. Concentration can also help you to avoid distractions and stay focused during your workout.

Mindfulness is another important technique that can help you to connect your mind and body during your Pilates bar workout. Mindfulness involves being aware of the present moment and fully engaging in the movement. By being mindful, you can improve your focus and concentration, which can help you to achieve better results. Mindfulness can also help you to stay motivated and avoid distractions during your workout.

Core Strength: Building a Strong Foundation for Your Body

Core strength is a crucial aspect of Pilates bar workout, as it forms the foundation for all other movements. A strong core not only improves your posture and balance, but also helps prevent injuries and enhances your overall physical performance. In this section, we'll explore the importance of core strength in Pilates bar workout and how you can build a strong foundation for your body.

First, let's define what we mean by the "core." Your core is not just your abdominal muscles, but also includes the muscles in your back, hips, and pelvis. These muscles work together to provide stability and support for your spine and pelvis, which are the center of your body.

In Pilates bar workout, you'll use your core muscles in every exercise, from basic movements like the Hundred to more advanced exercises like the Teaser. The focus on core strength allows you to move with control and precision, which is essential for getting the most out of your workout.

To build a strong core, it's important to start with the basics. Exercises like the Pilates plank, leg lifts, and pelvic tilts can help you develop the foundational strength you need to progress to more advanced movements. You should also incorporate exercises that target your back muscles, such as the Pilates swimming exercise, to ensure that you have balanced strength throughout your core.

One key aspect of building core strength in Pilates bar workout is learning to engage your deep core muscles, also known as your transverse abdominis. These muscles wrap around your spine like a corset, providing support and stability for your lower back. Engaging your deep core muscles can be challenging, but with practice, it becomes second nature.

To engage your deep core muscles, start by lying on your back with your knees bent and feet flat on the ground. Take a deep breath in, and as you exhale, imagine pulling your belly button in towards your spine. This engages your transverse abdominis and helps you stabilize your pelvis and lower back. Hold this engagement for a few seconds before releasing and repeating.

Another important aspect of core strength in Pilates bar workout is incorporating movements that challenge your stability and balance. Exercises like the Single Leg Stretch and the Corkscrew require you to maintain a stable core while moving your limbs, which can be a great way to build functional strength.

The Hundred

The Hundred is a classic Pilates exercise that targets the core muscles while also improving overall strength and endurance. To perform this exercise with the Pilates bar, begin by lying on your back with your legs in a tabletop position and your hands holding onto the bar, palms facing down. Engage your core and lift your head and shoulders off the mat.

Next, pump your arms up and down vigorously, while maintaining a steady breath pattern. Your arms should be pumping for 5 counts of inhales and 5 counts of exhales, for a total of 100 pumps. As you pump your arms, focus on keeping your core engaged and your spine in a neutral position.

To make the exercise more challenging, you can extend your legs out to a low diagonal position, keeping them hovering above the mat, or even straighten them out fully. Another option is to use resistance bands or additional weights on the Pilates bar to increase the intensity of the exercise.

The Criss-Cross

The Criss-Cross exercise is an effective Pilates bar workout that targets the abdominal muscles and helps build a strong core. Here's how to perform this exercise using the Pilates bar:

1. Lie down on your back on a mat or other comfortable surface. Hold the Pilates bar with both hands and extend your arms straight up towards the ceiling.
2. Lift your legs off the ground and bend your knees so that your calves are parallel to the floor. Your shins should be parallel to the Pilates bar.
3. Engage your core muscles and lift your head, neck, and shoulders off the ground. Keep your gaze forward, towards the ceiling.
4. Bring your right elbow towards your left knee, while simultaneously extending your right leg straight out, parallel to the floor. Keep your left leg bent.
5. Switch sides, bringing your left elbow towards your right knee, while extending your left leg straight out.
6. Continue alternating sides, twisting your torso as you bring each elbow towards the opposite knee.
7. Breathe deeply and rhythmically throughout the exercise, exhaling as you twist and inhaling as you return to the starting position.

To make the exercise more challenging, you can try increasing the speed or number of repetitions. You can also experiment with different grip positions on the Pilates bar to target different areas of your core muscles.

Planks

Planks are one of the most popular and effective exercises for building core strength and stability. The Pilates bar plank variation adds an extra challenge by incorporating the Pilates bar into the movement. This exercise targets the abs, lower back, shoulders, and arms, helping to build a strong and stable core.

To perform the Pilates bar plank variation, follow these steps:

1. Start by placing the Pilates bar on the ground in front of you, and come into a high plank position with your hands on the bar, shoulder-width apart.
2. Engage your core, and make sure your hips are in line with your shoulders and ankles. Your body should form a straight line from your head to your heels.
3. Hold this position for a few seconds, making sure to keep your core engaged and your back straight.
4. Slowly lower your body down towards the ground, bending your elbows to a 90-degree angle.
5. Hold this position for a few seconds, then push back up to the starting position.
6. Repeat for 10-15 repetitions, or as many as you can while maintaining good form.

Here are some tips to keep in mind when performing the Pilates bar plank variation:

- Keep your core engaged throughout the movement to maintain stability and prevent your hips from sagging.
- Keep your elbows close to your body when lowering down into the plank, rather than letting them flare out to the sides.
- Make sure your shoulders stay away from your ears, and avoid shrugging or tensing your neck muscles.

- Breathe deeply throughout the movement, inhaling as you lower down and exhaling as you push back up.

If you're new to the Pilates bar plank variation, start with a shorter hold time and fewer repetitions, gradually building up as your core strength improves.

The Teaser

To perform the Teaser, follow these steps:

1. Sit on your mat with your legs extended in front of you and your arms reaching towards the ceiling, holding the Pilates bar with both hands.
2. Engage your abdominal muscles and roll back onto your spine one vertebrae at a time.
3. Keep your arms reaching towards the ceiling and your legs hovering off the mat as you balance on your sacrum.
4. Slowly lower your legs towards the mat while simultaneously lowering your torso towards the mat, maintaining balance and control.
5. Return to the starting position by rolling up one vertebrae at a time until you're sitting upright again.

It's important to maintain proper form throughout the exercise to avoid straining your back or neck. Keep your shoulders relaxed and away from your ears, and maintain a long, straight spine throughout the exercise.

The Teaser can be modified to make it easier or more challenging, depending on your fitness level. If you're just starting out, you can bend your knees slightly to make the exercise easier. As you become more advanced, you can straighten your legs and lift them higher off the mat to make the exercise more challenging.

Single-Leg Circles

Single-Leg Circles is a fundamental Pilates Bar workout exercise that targets the core muscles, including the lower abs, hip flexors, and glutes. Here's how to perform the Single-Leg Circles exercise:

1. Begin by lying flat on your back with your arms by your sides and your legs extended straight out on the mat.
2. Hold the Pilates bar above your chest with both hands, making sure your arms are straight and your shoulders are relaxed.
3. Lift your right leg straight up towards the ceiling, keeping your left leg extended out on the mat.
4. Circle your right leg clockwise, drawing a large circle in the air with your toes, making sure to keep your hips stable and your lower back pressed into the mat.
5. After completing five circles clockwise, reverse the direction and perform five circles counterclockwise.
6. Lower your right leg back down to the mat and repeat the exercise with your left leg.

Some important things to keep in mind while performing Single-Leg Circles:

- Keep your core engaged throughout the exercise to help stabilize your hips and lower back.
- Make sure to keep your shoulders relaxed and your neck long.

- Focus on maintaining a steady, controlled movement, rather than rushing through the circles.
- If you experience any discomfort in your lower back or hips, make sure to modify the exercise or stop altogether.

Single-Leg Circles can be a challenging exercise, especially for beginners. It's important to start with a smaller circle and gradually work your way up to larger circles as your strength and stability improve. This exercise can also be modified by using a lighter resistance band or by performing the exercise without the Pilates bar altogether.

The Roll-Up

The Roll-Up is a classic Pilates exercise that targets the entire abdominal region, as well as the lower back and hip flexors.

To perform the Roll-Up, begin by lying on your back with your legs straight and your arms extended above your head, holding onto the Pilates bar with both hands. Take a deep breath in, and as you exhale, begin to roll your body up one vertebrae at a time, lifting your head, shoulders, and arms off the mat. Keep your arms straight and parallel to your legs as you roll up, and focus on using your abdominal muscles to control the movement.

When you reach a seated position, continue rolling forward until you are reaching towards your toes with your fingers. Take a deep breath in, and as you exhale, begin to roll your body back down one vertebrae at a time, keeping your arms straight and parallel to your legs. Lower your head, shoulders, and arms back down to the mat, and repeat for several repetitions.

To modify the Roll-Up, you can try bending your knees slightly and keeping your feet on the mat as you roll up and down, which can make the exercise more accessible for beginners or those with limited mobility. As you progress, you can gradually straighten your legs and work towards a full Roll-Up.

The Standing Oblique Twist

The standing oblique twist is a challenging Pilates bar workout that targets the oblique muscles, which are located on the sides of the abdominal muscles.

To perform the standing oblique twist, follow these steps:

1. Stand with your feet shoulder-width apart, and hold the Pilates bar with both hands, shoulder-width apart.
2. Engage your core muscles and keep your back straight.
3. Lift the Pilates bar above your head, with your arms fully extended.
4. Slowly twist your torso to the right, keeping your hips facing forward.
5. Pause for a moment at the end of the twist, then return to the starting position.
6. Repeat the twist to the left side, pausing at the end of the twist before returning to the starting position.
7. Repeat for several reps, or until you feel fatigued.

Inhale deeply through your nose as you lift the Pilates bar above your head, then exhale slowly as you twist to the right or left. It's important to start with a light weight Pilates bar and gradually increase the weight as you become more comfortable with the exercise.

CHAPTER 4: PILATES BAR WORKOUT EXERCISES

Barre Basics: Understanding the Importance of Barre Work in Pilates Bar Workout

Barre work is an essential component of Pilates bar workout, providing an intense full-body workout that improves strength, flexibility, and endurance. The use of a barre, or handrail, provides support and stability during exercises, enabling you to focus on proper alignment and form while challenging your muscles to work harder. In this section, we will explore the basics of barre work and how it benefits your Pilates bar workout.

The Origins of Barre Work

Barre work originated in the ballet world, where dancers used the barre to warm up and improve their technique. Over time, this practice evolved into a fitness trend that combines elements of ballet, Pilates, and strength training to create a unique and effective workout. Barre work has gained popularity in recent years due to its ability to tone muscles, improve posture, and increase flexibility without putting excessive stress on the joints.

The Importance of Barre Work in Pilates Bar Workout

In Pilates bar workout, barre work serves as a crucial foundation for building strength, balance, and endurance. Barre work exercises focus on strengthening the lower body, including the glutes, hips, thighs, and calves, while also engaging the core and upper body. By targeting these muscle groups, barre work improves stability, coordination, and overall body control.

One of the unique aspects of barre work in Pilates bar workout is the emphasis on small, controlled movements. These movements are designed to target specific muscle groups while also engaging the stabilizing muscles that support the joints. The use of the barre provides added support and stability, allowing you to focus on the quality of movement rather than the quantity. This approach leads to more significant improvements in muscle tone, endurance, and flexibility.

Barre work also benefits the cardiovascular system by increasing the heart rate and promoting blood flow throughout the body. The high-intensity nature of barre work means that it can burn calories and improve endurance, making it an effective addition to any fitness routine.

Basic Barre Work Exercises

Plie

The Pilates Bar workout Plie is a classic ballet move that is often incorporated into barre workouts. This exercise targets your lower body, particularly your thighs and glutes, while also engaging your core muscles. Here's how to perform the Pilates Bar workout Plie:

1. Start by standing with your feet wider than hip-width apart, toes pointed out at a 45-degree angle. Keep your spine long and your shoulders relaxed.
2. Hold onto your Pilates bar with both hands, palms facing down, and arms extended in front of you.
3. Slowly bend your knees and lower your body down, keeping your back straight and your weight on your heels. Aim to bring your thighs parallel to the ground.
4. Hold this position for a few seconds, then slowly rise back up to the starting position.
5. Repeat for 10-15 repetitions, or as many as you feel comfortable with.

Some key things to keep in mind while performing the Pilates Bar workout Plie:

- Make sure your knees are in line with your toes, and that they don't go past your toes. This helps prevent any strain on your knee joints.
- Engage your core muscles throughout the exercise to maintain stability and balance.
- Focus on keeping your weight on your heels to really target your glutes and thighs.
- If you're finding the exercise too challenging, try using a lighter resistance band or bar to start with.

Remember to breathe throughout the exercise. Inhale as you lower your body down, and exhale as you rise back up.

Releve

Releve is a classic ballet move that is incorporated into Pilates bar workout as a basic barre work exercise. Releve translates to "lifted" or "raised" in French, and that's exactly what you'll be doing with this exercise. Releve works the muscles in your feet, ankles, calves, and thighs, and it also helps improve your balance and posture. Here's how to perform Releve in Pilates bar workout:

1. Stand facing the barre with your feet parallel and hip-width apart. Place your hands lightly on the barre, keeping your shoulders relaxed.
2. Engage your core muscles and lift up onto the balls of your feet, keeping your heels lifted off the ground. Your weight should be evenly distributed between both feet.
3. Slowly lower your heels back down to the ground, keeping your movements controlled and smooth. Repeat this movement for several repetitions, feeling the burn in your calf muscles.
4. As you become more comfortable with the exercise, try lifting one foot off the ground and performing Releve on just one foot. Switch to the other foot after several repetitions.

To challenge yourself further, try performing Releve on a single leg with your arms extended out to the sides or overhead.

Tips for proper form:

- Keep your spine straight and your shoulders relaxed.
- Engage your core muscles to help you maintain your balance.
- Avoid locking your knees as you lift onto the balls of your feet.
- Make sure your weight is evenly distributed between both feet.

- Keep your movements slow and controlled to prevent any jerky motions.

The Arabesque

The Arabesque is a basic barre work exercise that targets the glutes, hamstrings, and core muscles. It is a challenging exercise that requires balance and control, but with practice, it can become a powerful addition to your Pilates Bar workout routine.

To perform the Arabesque, begin by standing at the barre with your feet parallel and hip-width apart. Place your right hand on the barre and lift your left leg behind you, keeping it straight and parallel to the floor. Your left arm should also be lifted in front of you, parallel to your left leg.

Next, engage your core muscles and lift your left leg higher, keeping it straight and parallel to the floor. At the same time, tilt your torso forward and lift your right arm behind you, parallel to your right leg. Your body should form a straight line from your fingertips to your toes.

Hold this position for a few seconds, focusing on maintaining balance and control. Then, lower your left leg back to the starting position and repeat the exercise on the opposite side.

It is important to maintain proper alignment throughout the exercise. Keep your shoulders relaxed and your hips level, and avoid arching your lower back. If you have difficulty maintaining balance, you can use the barre for support.

To make the Arabesque more challenging, you can add resistance by holding a small Pilates ball or using ankle weights. You can also incorporate pulsing movements to target the muscles even more.

Rond de jambes

Rond de jambes is a French term that translates to "round of the leg." It's a great exercise for strengthening and stretching the legs, particularly the hips and thighs. Here's how to perform the exercise:

1. Stand with your feet hip-distance apart, toes pointing forward, and hands on the barre for support.
2. Shift your weight to your left leg and lift your right leg slightly off the ground, keeping your foot pointed and your leg straight.
3. Begin circling your right leg in a clockwise direction, as if drawing a circle on the ground with your toes.
4. Make the circle as large as possible while keeping your hips stable and your standing leg straight.
5. Once you've completed a full circle, reverse the direction and circle your leg counterclockwise.
6. Complete 8-10 circles in each direction on one leg before switching to the other leg.

A few tips to keep in mind while performing Rond de jambes:

- Keep your hips level and stable throughout the exercise. Avoid tilting or shifting your pelvis.
- Keep your standing leg straight and engaged. Avoid locking your knee, but keep it firm.
- Keep your foot pointed throughout the exercise.

- Breathe deeply and rhythmically throughout the exercise.

Rond de jambes can be modified for different levels of ability. If you're just starting out, you can begin by making smaller circles and gradually increasing the size as you get stronger. If you're more advanced, you can try performing the exercise with ankle weights for added resistance.

Passe

The Passe exercise is a fundamental movement in barre work and is a great way to target and strengthen the legs, particularly the quads, hamstrings, and glutes. This exercise requires a Pilates bar and a stable surface, such as a wall or ballet barre, to hold onto for balance.

To perform the Passe exercise, follow these steps:

1. Begin by standing with your feet hip-width apart, facing the bar or wall. Place your hands on the bar for support.
2. Lift your right foot off the ground and bring it up to rest on the inside of your left knee. Your right knee should be bent and pointing out to the side.
3. Engage your core and glutes as you lift your left heel off the ground, rising up onto the ball of your foot.
4. Slowly lower your body back down, keeping your right foot in the Passe position.
5. Repeat for several repetitions on the right side before switching to the left.

Here are some tips to keep in mind while performing the Passe exercise:

- Keep your core engaged throughout the movement to help maintain balance and stability.
- Try to keep your standing leg straight and your knee pointing forward as much as possible.
- Focus on using your glutes and quads to lift your body up, rather than relying solely on your calf muscles.
- If you're struggling with balance, start by performing the exercise without lifting your heel off the ground, and gradually work your way up to the full movement.

Incorporating the Passe exercise into your Pilates Bar workout routine is a great way to target and strengthen your leg muscles while also improving balance and stability.

The Grand Battement

The Grand battement, also known as "big kick," Is a dynamic and elegant movement that requires strength, control, and flexibility. It involves lifting one leg off the ground and extending it fully to the front, side, or back, with pointed toes, while maintaining proper posture and alignment.

Here are the steps to perform the Grand battement:

1. Start in a standing position with your feet together and your arms resting at your sides. Keep your spine tall, your shoulders down, and your core engaged.
2. Shift your weight onto your right foot and lift your left leg off the ground slightly. Keep your left knee straight and your toes pointed.

3. Inhale deeply and as you exhale, kick your left leg forward, extending it fully from your hip, and reaching through your toes. Keep your standing leg stable and your upper body still.
4. Inhale again and lower your left leg back to the starting position with control. Repeat the movement to the side and then to the back.
5. Switch sides and perform the same movement with your right leg.

Here are some tips to keep in mind while performing the Grand battement:

- Keep your supporting leg straight and your foot firmly planted on the ground.
- Engage your glutes and hamstrings to lift and control your leg movements.
- Maintain proper posture by keeping your shoulders down, your chest open, and your core engaged.
- Avoid overextending your leg, which can lead to strain or injury. Instead, focus on maintaining control and precision in your movements.
- Take slow, deep breaths throughout the exercise to help you stay relaxed and focused.

The Grand battement is a great exercise for strengthening your legs, improving your balance and stability, and increasing your flexibility.

Tendus

Tendus is a fundamental exercise in Barre Work and is often used as a warm-up exercise to activate the leg muscles. This exercise helps to improve your balance, control, and coordination. Here's how to perform Tendus:

1. Start by standing in front of the Pilates Bar, with your feet hip-width apart and hands lightly resting on the bar.
2. Engage your core muscles by pulling your belly button towards your spine and standing tall with your shoulders relaxed.
3. Lift your right foot off the ground and point it to the front, keeping your toes on the ground.
4. Slowly drag your right foot along the floor to the side, while keeping your leg straight.
5. Return your right foot back to the starting position by pointing it to the front again.
6. Repeat this movement for 8-10 repetitions on the right side before switching to the left side.

Tips:

- Keep your supporting leg straight and your foot firmly planted on the ground throughout the exercise.
- Focus on lengthening your leg as you drag it along the floor to the side.
- Keep your torso stable and avoid leaning to the side.
- Work on your turnout by rotating your legs from your hips outward as you perform the exercise.

Upper Body Strengthening: Techniques for Building Arm, Shoulder, and Back Strength

In Pilates, a full-body workout is always emphasized, but it is also important to focus on specific areas that need improvement. The upper body is one of those areas that many people struggle with. The Pilates bar workout offers a variety of techniques that can help build arm, shoulder, and back strength. In this section, we will explore some of the most effective Pilates bar workout techniques for upper body strengthening.

The Upright Row

The upright row is a fantastic Pilates bar workout that targets the muscles in the shoulders, arms, and upper back.

To perform the upright row, you will need a Pilates bar and stand with your feet shoulder-width apart while holding the bar with an overhand grip. Your hands should be about shoulder-width apart with your arms extended in front of you.

From this starting position, exhale and slowly raise the bar towards your chin, keeping your elbows close to your body. As you lift the bar, focus on contracting the muscles in your shoulders, arms, and upper back. Make sure to keep your wrists straight and avoid using momentum to lift the bar.

Once the bar is level with your chin, pause for a moment, and then slowly lower it back down to the starting position while inhaling. Repeat this movement for several reps, focusing on maintaining proper form and engaging the target muscles.

When performing the upright row, there are a few important tips to keep in mind. First, it's crucial to maintain proper posture throughout the exercise. Keep your chest up, shoulders back, and avoid rounding your shoulders or hunching over the bar. This will help engage the correct muscles and prevent strain or injury.

Second, it's essential to use a weight that is appropriate for your fitness level. Starting with a lighter weight and gradually increasing as you become stronger is a good approach. Remember, form and technique are more important than the amount of weight lifted.

Back Row

The Pilates bar workout Back Row is an effective exercise for building strength in your upper back, shoulders, and arms.

Step-by-Step Guide to Performing the Pilates Bar Workout Back Row:

1. Begin by standing with your feet hip-width apart and knees slightly bent. Hold the Pilates bar with an overhand grip, shoulder-width apart, and palms facing down.
2. Keep your shoulders down and your back straight as you engage your core muscles.
3. Slowly bend your elbows and pull the bar towards your chest, keeping your elbows close to your body.
4. As you pull the bar towards your chest, squeeze your shoulder blades together, and focus on using your back muscles.
5. Hold the bar at chest level for a second and then slowly release back to the starting position.

6. Repeat for 8-12 reps, focusing on proper form and control throughout the movement.

Modifications:

- If you're a beginner, you can start with lighter resistance or perform the exercise without the Pilates bar. You can also perform the Back Row seated on a stability ball or bench to provide additional support.
- For advanced practitioners, you can increase the resistance of the Pilates bar or add a single-leg stance to challenge your balance and core stability.

Tips for Performing the Pilates Bar Workout Back Row:

- Keep your movements slow and controlled to ensure proper form and avoid injury.
- Focus on pulling the bar towards your chest with your back muscles rather than using your arms.
- Keep your elbows close to your body throughout the movement to maximize engagement of your upper back muscles.
- Engage your core muscles throughout the exercise to maintain stability and control.
- Avoid shrugging your shoulders or arching your back during the movement.

Triceps Extension

Triceps extensions are a great Pilates bar workout exercise to strengthen the muscles in the back of the arms. This exercise can be done with or without additional weights, depending on your fitness level and goals. Here's how to perform triceps extensions:

1. Start by standing with your feet shoulder-width apart, holding the Pilates bar with both hands behind your back.
2. Your hands should be close together and your palms facing down.
3. Keep your elbows close to your body and your shoulders relaxed.
4. Inhale and bend your elbows, lowering the Pilates bar behind your head.
5. Keep your upper arms close to your head and your shoulders relaxed.
6. Exhale and straighten your arms, lifting the Pilates bar back up to the starting position.
7. Repeat for several reps, then rest and repeat for another set.

Here are some tips to keep in mind when performing triceps extensions:

- If you are using additional weights, start with lighter weights and gradually increase as you build strength.
- Keep your core engaged throughout the exercise to maintain proper form.
- Focus on keeping your elbows close to your head and your shoulders relaxed.
- Avoid arching your back or letting your shoulders creep up towards your ears.

Rowing

Rowing targets the upper body, specifically the back muscles, shoulders, and arms.

Here's how to do it:

1. Start by standing with your feet shoulder-width apart, holding the Pilates bar in front of you with an overhand grip, palms facing down.
2. Keep your arms straight and extend the Pilates bar in front of you.
3. Keeping your arms straight, slowly lift the Pilates bar towards your chest, pulling your elbows back towards your body.
4. As you lift the Pilates bar, squeeze your shoulder blades together.
5. Hold the Pilates bar at chest level for a few seconds, then slowly lower it back down to the starting position.
6. Repeat for several reps, focusing on keeping your movements slow and controlled.

Tips:

- Make sure to keep your shoulders relaxed throughout the exercise. Do not shrug your shoulders up towards your ears.
- As you lift the Pilates bar towards your chest, make sure to keep your elbows close to your body. This will help engage the muscles in your back and shoulders more effectively.
- Exhale as you lift the Pilates bar towards your chest, and inhale as you lower it back down.
- To increase the difficulty of the exercise, try holding the Pilates bar at chest level for a few seconds before lowering it back down.

The Lateral Raise

The lateral raise is a classic exercise that targets the shoulders and helps to build shoulder strength and stability.

Here's how to perform the lateral raise exercise with a Pilates bar:

1. Start by standing with your feet shoulder-width apart, with your Pilates bar in front of you at waist height.
2. Grab the bar with an overhand grip, keeping your palms facing downwards, and your hands shoulder-width apart.
3. Engage your core and keep your back straight as you raise the bar out to the side, keeping your arms straight and parallel to the floor.
4. Make sure you keep your shoulders down and relaxed, and focus on engaging your shoulder muscles as you lift the bar.
5. Hold the position for a few seconds, then slowly lower the bar back down to your starting position.
6. Repeat for the desired number of repetitions.

You can also vary the intensity of the exercise by using a heavier or lighter Pilates bar.

Shoulder Press

To perform the Shoulder Press in Pilates bar workout, follow these steps:

1. Begin by standing with your feet hip-width apart and holding the Pilates bar with both hands, palms facing forward. Your arms should be extended straight up above your head, with the bar resting on your shoulders.

2. Inhale and engage your core muscles, keeping your spine straight and your shoulders down away from your ears.
3. Exhale and press the bar straight up towards the ceiling, extending your arms fully. Keep your elbows close to your head and your wrists straight.
4. Inhale and lower the bar back down to your shoulders, keeping your arms close to your body and your wrists straight.
5. Repeat the movement for 10-15 reps, focusing on maintaining proper form and breathing throughout the exercise.

Tips for performing the Shoulder Press:

- Make sure to engage your core muscles throughout the exercise to maintain proper form and stability.
- Keep your shoulders down away from your ears and your spine straight to prevent any strain or injury.
- Use a light to moderate weight for the Pilates bar to start with, and gradually increase the weight as your strength improves.

Lower Body Sculpting: Exercises for Developing Strong Legs, Glutes, and Hips

In this section, we will discuss how Pilates bar workouts can help you achieve strong and toned legs, glutes, and hips, as well as some effective exercises to include in your routine.

Plie Squats

This exercise is based on the traditional plie movement used in ballet, but modified for Pilates bar workouts to increase resistance and intensity.

Step-by-Step Guide to Performing Pilates Bar Workout Plie Squats:

1. Start by standing with your feet shoulder-width apart, with your toes pointing outwards at a 45-degree angle. Hold the Pilates bar with both hands, keeping your arms straight and parallel to the ground.
2. Engage your core muscles, and slowly lower your body down into a squat position. Keep your back straight and your knees in line with your toes.
3. As you lower your body, simultaneously raise the Pilates bar up towards your chest. Your elbows should be pointing outwards, away from your body.
4. Once you have lowered your body as far as possible, hold the position for a few seconds, then slowly raise yourself back up to the starting position. As you do so, lower the Pilates bar back down to its original position.
5. Repeat this movement for several repetitions, aiming to perform at least 10-12 squats in a row.

Tips for Effective Performance:

- Focus on your form: Proper form is essential for getting the most out of any Pilates bar workout exercise. Make sure to keep your back straight and your core engaged throughout the exercise, and be careful not to let your knees extend over your toes.
- Use controlled movements: Pilates bar workouts are all about controlled, deliberate movements. Make sure to lower yourself into the squat position slowly and smoothly, and avoid sudden, jerky movements.
- Keep the bar stable: As you perform the exercise, make sure to keep the Pilates bar stable and under control. Don't swing it around or use momentum to lift your body up from the squat position.
- Adjust the resistance as needed: If you find that the exercise is too easy or too difficult, you can adjust the resistance of the Pilates bar by adding or removing weights. Start with a lighter weight if you are a beginner, and gradually increase the weight as you become stronger and more comfortable with the exercise.

Incorporate variations: Once you have mastered the basic plie squat, you can incorporate variations to increase the challenge and target different muscle groups. For example, you can try holding the squat position for longer periods of time, or adding a pulse at the bottom of the movement to really engage your glutes and thighs.

Hip Bridge

This is an excellent exercise for developing strong glutes, hips, and lower back muscles. This exercise primarily targets the glutes, but it also works the lower back and hips.

To perform the Pilates bar workout hip bridge, follow these steps:

1. Lie on your back on a mat with your knees bent and feet flat on the floor. Place the Pilates bar across your hip bones and hold it in place with your hands.
2. Inhale and engage your core muscles by drawing your navel in towards your spine.
3. Exhale and slowly lift your hips up towards the ceiling, squeezing your glutes and pressing your feet firmly into the floor.
4. Pause at the top of the movement and inhale.
5. Exhale and slowly lower your hips back down to the starting position, keeping your core engaged throughout the movement.
6. Repeat this exercise for 10-12 repetitions, or as many as you can comfortably perform with good form.

Here are a few things to keep in mind when performing the Pilates bar workout hip bridge:

- Make sure to keep your feet flat on the floor throughout the movement, and press them firmly into the ground for stability.
- Keep your shoulders and upper back flat on the mat throughout the movement, and avoid letting them lift off the ground.
- Focus on squeezing your glutes at the top of the movement to maximize the activation of your glute muscles.

- Avoid arching your lower back excessively, as this can put unnecessary strain on your back muscles.
- Breathe deeply and rhythmically throughout the exercise, inhaling as you prepare for the movement and exhaling as you lift your hips.

Bridge Lifts

Steps for Performing Pilates Bar Workout Bridge Lifts

1. Start by lying on your back on a mat with your knees bent and feet flat on the ground. Place your Pilates bar across your hips, holding it with your palms facing down.
2. Make sure your feet are hip-width apart and your toes are pointing straight ahead.
3. Take a deep breath in and, as you exhale, lift your hips off the ground, pressing the Pilates bar towards the ceiling. Keep your arms straight and your hands firmly holding the bar.
4. Hold the position for a few seconds, then inhale and slowly lower your hips back down to the mat.
5. Repeat the exercise for 10-15 repetitions.

Tips for Performing Pilates Bar Workout Bridge Lifts

- Focus on squeezing your glutes and engaging your core muscles as you lift your hips off the ground. This will help you maintain proper form and prevent injury.
- Keep your feet firmly planted on the ground throughout the exercise. This will help you maintain balance and stability.
- If you find the exercise too challenging, you can perform it without the Pilates bar until you build up your strength.

- As you lift your hips, make sure your knees stay in line with your ankles. Avoid letting your knees splay out to the sides, as this can strain your hip muscles.
- Keep your shoulders relaxed and avoid tensing them up towards your ears.

The Side Leg Lift

The side leg lift is an effective Pilates bar workout exercise for sculpting your outer thighs, hips, and glutes. This exercise also helps to improve your balance and stability, making it a great addition to your lower body workout routine. Here's how to perform this exercise correctly:

Step 1: Preparation

Begin by standing with your feet hip-width apart, and your Pilates bar resting against your hips. Keep your core engaged and your shoulders relaxed.

Step 2: Movement

Slowly lift your right leg out to the side while keeping your toes pointed forward. Be sure to keep your hips level and your standing leg slightly bent. As you lift your leg, inhale deeply and engage your glutes and outer thigh muscles.

Step 3: Hold and Lower

Hold your leg up for a few seconds and then lower it back down to the starting position while exhaling. Repeat the exercise on the same side for 10-12 reps before switching to the other leg.

Tips for Proper Form:

- Keep your torso upright and avoid leaning to one side as you lift your leg.
- Be sure to engage your core muscles throughout the exercise to maintain your balance.
- Don't let your lifted leg drop too low as you lower it down to avoid overstretching your hip.
- Keep your standing leg slightly bent throughout the exercise to maintain proper alignment.

Modifications:

If you're just starting with Pilates bar workouts, you may find it challenging to lift your leg high without losing your balance. In that case, you can try a modified version of the side leg lift by placing your hand on a nearby wall or barre to help you maintain your balance. Additionally, you can also use a resistance band around your thighs to add extra resistance and increase the difficulty of the exercise.

Squat Jumps

Squat jumps are an excellent Pilates bar workout exercise for building lower body strength and improving cardiovascular endurance. This exercise is a combination of a squat and a jump, making it a great compound exercise that targets multiple muscle groups at once. Here is a step-by-step guide on how to perform squat jumps correctly:

Step 1: Start by standing with your feet hip-width apart and your toes pointing forward. Hold the Pilates bar with both hands in front of your chest, elbows bent, and palms facing down.

Step 2: Lower your hips down and back into a squat position, keeping your knees behind your toes and your weight in your heels. Make sure to keep your chest lifted and your spine neutral.

Step 3: Once you have reached the bottom of your squat, jump up explosively, extending your legs and pushing through your feet. As you jump, raise the Pilates bar overhead and straighten your arms impact

Step 4: Land softly back into your starting position, lowering your arms and bending your knees to absorb the impact.

Step 5: Repeat the exercise for a set number of reps or for a set amount of time, depending on your workout goals.

To perform side lunges with the Pilates bar, follow these steps:

- Begin by standing with your feet hip-width apart, holding the Pilates bar with both hands in front of your body at chest height.
- Take a wide step to the right, keeping your toes pointing forward and your left foot firmly planted on the ground.
- As you step to the side, bend your right knee and hinge forward at the hips, keeping your back straight and your chest lifted. Your weight should be in your right heel.
- Press through your right heel to return to standing, and then repeat on the other side.
- Aim for 10-12 repetitions on each side, or as many as you can perform with proper form.

When performing side lunges with the Pilates bar, there are a few things to keep in mind to ensure proper form and maximum effectiveness:

- Keep your chest lifted and your shoulders down and back throughout the movement.
- Engage your core muscles to help stabilize your body and maintain balance.
- Make sure that your knee is tracking over your toes, rather than collapsing inward or outward.
- Keep your weight in your heels to engage your glutes and hamstrings.
- Don't let your opposite foot lift off the ground as you lunge to the side.

Full-Body Workouts: Combining Upper and Lower Body Exercises for Total-Body Transformation

While it's great to focus on specific areas of the body, such as the core or the legs, incorporating full-body workouts can provide even more significant benefits. Full-body Pilates Bar workouts combine both upper and lower body exercises to create a total-body transformation that leaves you feeling strong, energized, and balanced.

The Plank with Knee Tuck

The Plank with Knee Tuck is a challenging and effective Pilates Bar workout that targets the entire body, with a focus on the core and upper body. This exercise combines the plank, which is an excellent total body exercise, with a knee tuck, which engages the core and lower body. Here is a step-by-step guide on how to perform the Pilates Bar Workout Plank with Knee Tuck:

Step 1: Begin in a plank position with your hands shoulder-width apart on the Pilates Bar and your toes on the ground, hip-width apart. Your body should be in a straight line from your head to your heels, with your core engaged and your shoulders over your wrists.

Step 2: Keeping your body straight and your core engaged, lift your right knee towards your chest.

Step 3: Return your right leg to the plank position.

Step 4: Repeat the knee tuck with your left leg.

Step 5: Continue alternating knee tucks for a total of 10 repetitions (5 each leg).

Tips for Performing the Pilates Bar Workout Plank with Knee Tuck:

- Engage your core muscles throughout the entire exercise. This will help stabilize your body and prevent your lower back from sagging.
- Keep your shoulders over your wrists and your neck in line with your spine. Avoid looking up or dropping your head.
- Focus on your breath. Inhale as you bring your knee towards your chest, and exhale as you return your leg to the plank position.
- Make sure your Pilates Bar is securely fastened and stable before beginning the exercise.
- Start with 5-10 repetitions and gradually increase the number as you become stronger and more comfortable with the exercise.

Squat with Overhead Press

The Pilates Bar Workout Squat with Overhead Press is a compound exercise that targets multiple muscle groups in the body. It primarily works the lower body muscles like the glutes, quads, and hamstrings while also engaging the upper body muscles like the shoulders, triceps, and core.

To perform the Pilates Bar Workout Squat with Overhead Press, follow these steps:

1. Start by standing with your feet hip-width apart and your toes pointing forward. Hold the Pilates bar with both hands and rest it on your shoulders.
2. Inhale and squat down, keeping your back straight and your knees behind your toes. Lower your body until your thighs are parallel to the ground.
3. Exhale and stand up, pressing the Pilates bar overhead until your arms are fully extended.
4. Inhale and lower the Pilates bar back to your shoulders.
5. Repeat the squat and overhead press for a total of 10-12 reps.

Here are some tips to keep in mind while performing the Pilates Bar Workout Squat with Overhead Press:

- Make sure to keep your back straight throughout the exercise. Avoid leaning forward or rounding your spine.
- Keep your knees behind your toes while squatting to prevent any strain on your knee joints.

- Engage your core muscles to maintain stability and balance throughout the movement.
- Exhale as you press the Pilates bar overhead and inhale as you lower it back down to your shoulders.
- Gradually increase the weight of the Pilates bar as you become stronger and more comfortable with the exercise.

Single-Leg Deadlifts With Row

To perform the exercise:

1. Stand with your feet hip-width apart and hold the Pilates bar in both hands, with your palms facing down.
2. Shift your weight onto your left foot and lift your right leg off the ground, extending it behind you.
3. Hinge forward at your hips, keeping your spine straight, and lower the Pilates bar towards the ground.
4. At the same time, lift your right leg higher, keeping it in line with your torso.
5. Once you reach your maximum range of motion, pause for a moment, then squeeze your glutes and engage your core to lift your torso back up to a standing position.
6. As you lift your torso, pull the Pilates bar towards your chest, bending your elbows and keeping them close to your sides.
7. Lower the Pilates bar back down towards the ground as you hinge forward again and lift your right leg off the ground.
8. Repeat the exercise for the desired number of reps, then switch sides and repeat with your left leg.

Tips for proper form:

- Keep your spine straight and your shoulders relaxed throughout the exercise.
- Engage your core and squeeze your glutes to maintain balance and stability.
- Avoid arching your back or rounding your shoulders.
- Focus on your breath, inhaling as you lift your torso and exhaling as you hinge forward.

Single-Leg Deadlifts with Row

The single-leg deadlift with row is an excellent full-body exercise that targets multiple muscle groups, including the legs, back, and core. It requires a Pilates bar and weights.

Here's how to perform this exercise:

1. Start by standing tall with your feet hip-width apart, holding a Pilates bar in front of your thighs with an overhand grip.
2. Shift your weight to your left foot and lift your right foot off the floor, balancing on your left leg.
3. Slowly hinge forward at the hips, keeping your back straight and your core engaged. As you hinge forward, lift the Pilates bar towards your chest, keeping your elbows close to your sides.
4. Lower the Pilates bar and hinge forward until your torso is parallel to the floor, and your right leg extends behind you.
5. Pause briefly and then pull the Pilates bar towards your chest, keeping your elbows close to your sides.
6. Lower the Pilates bar and return to the starting position.
7. Repeat on the opposite leg.

Here are some tips to keep in mind when performing the single-leg deadlift with row:

- Keep your core engaged throughout the exercise to help maintain balance and stability.
- Keep your back straight and your shoulders relaxed to avoid strain on your lower back.
- If you're new to the exercise, start with a light weight and gradually increase as you get stronger and more comfortable with the movement.
- Focus on controlling the movement, rather than rushing through it, to maximize its effectiveness.

The Reverse Lunge with Bicep Curl

To perform the reverse lunge with bicep curl:

1. Begin by standing with your feet hip-width apart, holding the Pilates bar in both hands with an underhand grip. Keep your elbows close to your sides and your shoulders relaxed.
2. Step your left foot back, bending both knees to lower your body down into a lunge. Keep your front knee directly over your ankle, and your back knee hovering just above the ground.
3. As you lower down into the lunge, curl the Pilates bar up towards your shoulders, bending your elbows and keeping them close to your sides. Pause for a moment at the bottom of the lunge, holding the Pilates bar steady.
4. Press through your front heel to stand back up, straightening both legs and lowering the Pilates bar back down to your sides.

5. Repeat the lunge on the opposite side, stepping your right foot back and curling the Pilates bar up towards your shoulders.
6. Continue alternating sides, performing 8-12 repetitions on each leg for a total of 16-24 reps.

When performing the reverse lunge with bicep curl, it's important to keep your core engaged and your back straight, with your shoulders relaxed and your chest lifted. Make sure to lower down into the lunge slowly and with control, and avoid letting your front knee collapse inward or your back knee touch the ground. Keep your gaze forward and your breathing steady throughout the exercise.

To modify the exercise, you can perform the reverse lunge without the Pilates bar, or use lighter weights if the Pilates bar feels too heavy. You can also reduce the range of motion in the lunge if you feel any discomfort in your knees or hips.

The Chest Fly with Bridge

To perform the chest fly with bridge, follow these steps:

1. Start by lying on your back with your knees bent and feet flat on the ground. Hold the Pilates bar with both hands, palms facing up, and extend your arms straight up over your chest.
2. Inhale as you lower the bar down towards your chest, keeping your elbows slightly bent and your arms in line with your shoulders.
3. Exhale as you lift the bar back up to the starting position, engaging your chest muscles.

4. As you lift the bar, also lift your hips off the ground to form a bridge position. Keep your shoulders and upper back on the ground and engage your glutes and core to hold the position.
5. Inhale as you lower your hips back down to the ground, keeping the bar lifted above your chest.
6. Repeat for 10-12 reps, focusing on keeping your movements slow and controlled.

Keep your core engaged throughout the movement to protect your lower back and maintain a neutral spine. Avoid letting your elbows flare out to the sides and keep your wrists in a neutral position to prevent any strain on your wrists or shoulders.

To modify this exercise, you can perform the chest fly without the bridge or lower the intensity by using a lighter resistance on the Pilates bar. To increase the intensity, you can use a heavier resistance or add a pause at the bottom of the movement to further engage your chest muscles.

The Standing Wood Chop

The standing wood chop is a dynamic and challenging exercise that targets the entire body, with a focus on the core, legs, and upper body. Here's how to perform the standing wood chop with a Pilates bar:

1. Stand with your feet hip-width apart, holding the Pilates bar with both hands. Hold the bar at shoulder height, with your arms fully extended and your palms facing down.
2. Take a deep breath and engage your core muscles. Shift your weight to your left foot and pivot on your left foot, rotating

your torso to the right. Your right foot should pivot slightly as well, but keep it planted on the ground.

3. As you rotate your torso to the right, bring the Pilates bar diagonally down and across your body, ending with the bar outside your left knee.

4. Exhale and contract your core muscles as you reverse the movement, bringing the Pilates bar back up and across your body to the starting position. At the same time, pivot on your left foot and rotate your torso to the left.

5. Repeat the exercise for 10-12 repetitions on one side, then switch to the other side.

Here are a few tips to keep in mind when performing the standing wood chop:

- Start with a lighter weight Pilates bar until you feel comfortable with the movement and can maintain proper form.

- Keep your core engaged throughout the exercise to protect your lower back and maximize the benefits to your core muscles.

- Control the movement and avoid using momentum to swing the Pilates bar. This will help you target the muscles more effectively and prevent injury.

- Focus on rotating your torso as you pivot on your feet. This will help you engage your obliques and improve your rotational stability.

Pile Squats with Overhead Press

This exercise is a great way to challenge yourself and achieve a total-body transformation.

To perform the pile squat with overhead press, follow these steps:

1. Start by standing with your feet wider than hip-width apart, with your toes pointed slightly outward.
2. Hold the Pilates bar with both hands, resting it on your shoulders.
3. Lower your body down into a squat position, keeping your chest up and your back straight. Make sure your knees are in line with your toes.
4. From the squat position, push through your heels to stand up, lifting the Pilates bar overhead.
5. Lower the Pilates bar back to your shoulders as you lower your body back down into the squat position.
6. Repeat the movement for 10-15 reps.

Here are some tips to keep in mind when performing the pile squat with overhead press:

- Make sure to keep your chest up and your back straight throughout the entire movement.
- As you push through your heels to stand up, make sure to engage your glutes and core.
- When lifting the Pilates bar overhead, make sure to fully extend your arms and keep the bar directly over your head.
- When lowering the Pilates bar back to your shoulders, make sure to control the movement and avoid swinging the bar.

CHAPTER 5: ADVANCED PILATES BAR WORKOUT TECHNIQUES

Balancing Act: The Art of Balance in Pilates Bar Workout

Balance is a crucial component of any exercise program. It helps improve stability, coordination, and posture, which can lead to better overall fitness and reduced risk of injuries. In Pilates bar workout, balance is particularly important as it helps to engage the core muscles, enhance proprioception, and increase body awareness. In this section, we will explore the art of balance in Pilates bar workout, why it is essential, and techniques to improve balance.

Why Balance Is Important in Pilates Bar Workout

In Pilates bar workout, balance is critical for several reasons. Firstly, it is essential for engaging the core muscles. The core muscles are responsible for stabilizing the spine and pelvis during movements. When you perform exercises that challenge your balance, your core muscles have to work harder to keep you stable. As a result, you get a more effective core workout.

Secondly, balance helps to enhance proprioception. Proprioception is the ability to sense the position and movement of your body in space. Good proprioception allows you to perform movements with accuracy, speed, and control. When you improve your balance, you also improve your proprioception.

Finally, balance training can increase body awareness. When you focus on maintaining balance, you become more aware of your body and how it moves. This increased body awareness can help you identify areas of weakness or imbalance, which can then be addressed through targeted exercises.

Techniques to Improve Balance in Pilates Bar Workout

Here are some effective techniques to improve balance in Pilates bar workout:

Start with a stable base

Before attempting any balance exercises, it is essential to start with a stable base. This means ensuring that your feet are firmly planted on the ground and your weight is evenly distributed. Take a few moments to stand in a neutral position with your feet hip-distance apart, and focus on grounding your feet into the floor.

Use a stable support

If you are new to balance training, or if you have balance issues, it is helpful to use a stable support. This can be a wall, a chair, or even a Pilates bar. Using a support allows you to focus on maintaining balance without worrying about falling over. As you improve, you can gradually reduce the amount of support you use.

Practice one-legged balance exercises

One-legged balance exercises are a great way to improve balance and engage the core muscles. Start with simple exercises such as standing on one leg and gradually progress to more challenging exercises such as one-legged squats or lunges. Make sure to keep your core engaged and your gaze fixed on a stable point in front of you.

Try balance equipment

There are several pieces of equipment that can be used to improve balance in Pilates bar workout. These include balance balls, balance boards, and foam rollers. Using these pieces of equipment can add an extra challenge to your balance exercises and help to improve proprioception.

Incorporate balance challenges into your Pilates bar workout

Incorporating balance challenges into your Pilates bar workout can help to improve balance while also providing a full-body workout. Exercises such as single-leg squats with a Pilates bar or one-legged bridge poses can challenge your balance and engage multiple muscle groups at the same time.

The Single Leg Squat with Leg Lift

The single leg squat with leg lift is a challenging yet rewarding Pilates bar workout exercise that helps improve balance and stability while strengthening the lower body. Here's how to perform it and everything you need to know:

1. Set up your equipment: Start by attaching your resistance band to the Pilates bar at a low level. Stand with your feet hip-width apart and place the loop of the resistance band around your right foot. Hold the Pilates bar with both hands at chest height.
2. Lift your leg: Shift your weight onto your left foot and lift your right leg off the ground, keeping it straight and parallel to the floor. Engage your core muscles to maintain balance.
3. Squat: Slowly lower yourself into a squat position, keeping your left knee bent and your back straight. Try to keep your weight centered over your left foot.
4. Lift your leg again: As you rise back up to a standing position, lift your right leg up towards the ceiling, maintaining the straight line from your foot to your head.
5. Repeat: Do 10-15 reps on one side before switching to the other leg.

Tips:

- If you're having trouble balancing, try focusing on a fixed point in front of you or engaging your core muscles more.
- Make sure to keep your knee tracking over your toes as you squat to avoid any strain on your knee joint.
- You can also adjust the resistance level of the band to make the exercise easier or more challenging.

The Single-Leg Squat with Overhead Press

To perform the Single-Leg Squat with Overhead Press, follow these steps:

1. Start by standing with your feet hip-distance apart and holding the Pilates bar in both hands, resting it on your shoulders.
2. Shift your weight onto your left foot and lift your right foot off the ground.
3. Engage your core and maintain good posture, keeping your shoulders down and back.
4. Lower yourself into a squat position by bending your left knee, keeping your right leg lifted off the ground.
5. As you squat, raise the Pilates bar above your head until your arms are fully extended.
6. Pause for a moment and then return to the starting position by straightening your left leg and lowering the Pilates bar back down to your shoulders.
7. Repeat the exercise on the other side by shifting your weight onto your right foot and lifting your left foot off the ground.

Here are some key points to keep in mind when performing the Single-Leg Squat with Overhead Press:

- Keep your weight centered over the middle of your foot.
- Engage your core and maintain good posture throughout the exercise.
- Focus on keeping your knee in line with your toes as you lower yourself into the squat position.

- Keep your shoulders down and back, and avoid shrugging them up toward your ears.
- As you raise the Pilates bar above your head, be sure to fully extend your arms.
- Keep your gaze forward and maintain your balance by engaging your core muscles.

The Balancing Lunge

The Balancing Lunge is an excellent exercise for working on balance and coordination while also toning the legs and glutes. Here's a step-by-step guide on how to perform the Balancing Lunge using a Pilates bar:

1. Begin by standing with your feet together and holding the Pilates bar at chest height with both hands.
2. Step forward with your right foot, keeping your weight in your front heel and your back toe.
3. Bend your front knee to a 90-degree angle, keeping your back leg straight and your back heel lifted off the ground.
4. As you lunge forward, tilt your upper body forward slightly, keeping the Pilates bar close to your chest.
5. Hold the position for a few seconds, then push off with your front foot to return to the starting position.
6. Repeat on the other side, stepping forward with your left foot and lunging down.
7. Keep your movements slow and controlled, focusing on your balance and stability throughout the exercise.

Tips for performing the Balancing Lunge:

- Start with a light Pilates bar or no weight at all until you feel comfortable with the movement.
- Keep your core engaged throughout the exercise to help with balance and stability.
- If you're having trouble balancing, focus on a fixed point in front of you to help stabilize your gaze.
- Be sure to keep your knee in line with your ankle and don't let it extend over your toes.
- If you have knee pain or injury, take caution when performing this exercise and stop if you feel any discomfort.

Standing Leg Circles

Here's a step-by-step guide on how to perform the standing leg circles correctly:

1. Begin by standing upright with your feet hip-distance apart, holding the Pilates bar in front of you at chest height with both hands. Keep your shoulders relaxed and your core engaged.
2. Shift your weight onto your left foot and lift your right foot off the ground, flexing your foot.
3. Slowly begin to draw a large circle with your right leg, moving it clockwise. Keep your leg straight, and try to keep your hips as still as possible.
4. Once you've completed a full circle, reverse the direction and move your leg counterclockwise.
5. Repeat for 8-10 repetitions on one leg, then switch to the other leg and repeat the same movement.

Here are some tips to keep in mind when performing the standing leg circles:

- Keep your standing leg slightly bent and your knee soft to avoid locking your knee and to maintain balance.
- Focus on keeping your hips level and stable throughout the exercise. You can use a mirror to check your form and make sure you're not tilting to one side.
- Keep your core engaged throughout the exercise to help maintain your balance and stability.
- Take deep breaths and try to relax your shoulders and upper body as much as possible.
- You can modify the exercise by holding onto a stable surface such as a chair or a wall for balance.

The Side Plank with Arm Reach

Here's how to perform this exercise:

1. Start in a side plank position with your right hand on the Pilates bar and your feet stacked on top of each other. Your left hand should be on your hip.
2. Engage your core muscles and lift your hips off the ground, so your body forms a straight line from your head to your feet.
3. Reach your left arm up towards the ceiling, keeping it in line with your shoulder.
4. Hold this position for a few seconds, then return to the starting position.
5. Repeat on the other side.

Here are some tips to keep in mind while performing this exercise:

- Make sure to keep your body in a straight line throughout the exercise. Avoid letting your hips sag towards the ground or lifting them too high.
- Engage your core muscles throughout the exercise to maintain proper form and balance.
- Keep your shoulders relaxed and away from your ears.
- Focus on your breathing. Inhale as you lower your body down, and exhale as you lift it up.

Warrior III

To perform the Warrior III Pilates bar workout exercise, follow these steps:

1. Start by standing with your feet hip-width apart, facing the Pilates bar. Place your hands on the bar, shoulder-width apart.
2. Take a deep breath in and exhale while slowly lifting your right leg off the ground, keeping it straight behind you.
3. Keep your arms straight as you hinge forward at the hips, extending your right leg back and lifting it to hip height.
4. At the same time, reach your left arm forward, parallel to the ground, and your right arm back, also parallel to the ground.
5. Engage your core muscles and maintain a straight line from your head to your right heel.
6. Hold this position for a few breaths, then inhale and slowly lower your right leg to the ground.
7. Repeat the same movement with your left leg.

Now that you know how to perform the Warrior III Pilates bar workout exercise, let's take a closer look at some tips to help you perform it correctly and safely:

- Keep your hips square: Make sure that your hips are level and facing the ground. Avoid rotating them to the side.
- Engage your core: Your core muscles play a crucial role in this exercise, as they help to stabilize your body and maintain balance.
- Focus on your breathing: Inhale deeply before you start, and exhale as you lift your leg and hinge forward. Focus on maintaining a steady breath throughout the exercise.
- Keep your shoulders relaxed: Avoid shrugging your shoulders or tensing your neck muscles. Instead, keep your shoulders down and away from your ears.
- Keep your gaze forward: Look straight ahead to help maintain your balance and focus.

The Tree Pose

The Tree Pose is a classic yoga pose that has been adapted for use with the Pilates bar. This pose is excellent for improving balance, coordination, and core stability, and can be done by anyone, regardless of fitness level or experience with Pilates.

Here's how to perform the Tree Pose with a Pilates bar:

1. Start by standing with your feet together and your Pilates bar at your side.

2. Place your right foot on your left inner thigh, just above the knee. Your foot should be pressing into your thigh, and your knee should be pointing out to the side.
3. Slowly raise your Pilates bar up over your head, holding it with both hands.
4. Focus on your balance and stability as you hold the pose for several breaths.
5. Release the pose and repeat on the other side.

It's essential to maintain good form and alignment while doing the Tree Pose with a Pilates bar. Here are some tips to help you get the most out of this exercise:

- Keep your core engaged throughout the pose. This will help you maintain your balance and stability.
- Focus on your breath as you hold the pose. Inhale deeply through your nose, filling your lungs with air, and exhale slowly through your mouth.
- Keep your shoulders relaxed and down, away from your ears. This will help you avoid tension in your upper body.
- If you're having trouble balancing, try focusing your gaze on a stationary object in front of you, such as a wall or a piece of furniture.

Pushing the Limits: Advanced Techniques for Experienced Practitioners

For experienced Pilates practitioners, it can be easy to fall into a routine and become comfortable with the same exercises. However, pushing the limits and incorporating advanced techniques can help break through plateaus and lead to even greater results.

Below are some advanced Pilates bar workout techniques for experienced practitioners:

One-Legged Squat with Knee Raise

This move is not for beginners, so make sure you have a solid foundation of Pilates bar work before attempting it.

Here's how to perform the one-legged squat with knee raise:

1. Stand with your feet hip-width apart, holding the Pilates bar at shoulder height with both hands. Your palms should be facing forward.
2. Shift your weight onto your left leg and lift your right foot off the ground. Hold your right knee up in front of your body.
3. Begin to lower your body down into a squat position, keeping your weight in your left heel and your chest lifted. Aim to get your left thigh parallel to the ground.
4. As you lower down, raise your right leg straight out in front of you, extending it until it is parallel to the ground.
5. Hold this position for a beat or two, then return to the starting position, lowering your right foot back down to the ground and standing up straight.

6. Repeat the movement, this time shifting your weight onto your right leg and lifting your left foot off the ground.

Some tips to keep in mind:

- As with any Pilates bar exercise, it's important to engage your core muscles throughout the movement to maintain stability and control.
- Make sure your knee is tracking over your ankle as you lower down into the squat position. Avoid letting your knee cave inward or pushing it past your toes.
- Keep your gaze forward and your chest lifted throughout the movement. This will help you maintain good posture and balance.
- If you find this exercise too challenging at first, you can practice it with a chair or wall nearby to use for support. You can also try doing it without the Pilates bar to start, and gradually work up to incorporating the bar into the movement.

Hanging Leg Lifts

This exercise primarily targets the lower abs, hip flexors, and quads.

Here's how to perform the hanging leg lifts using the Pilates bar:

1. Begin by finding a secure pull-up bar that can support your weight. Grasp the bar with an overhand grip and hang with your arms fully extended. Your palms should be facing away from your body, and your shoulders should be relaxed and down away from your ears.

2. Engage your core muscles, and use your lower abs to lift your legs up toward the Pilates bar. Keep your legs straight and your toes pointed.
3. Lift your legs as high as you can without swinging or using momentum. Hold the position briefly at the top of the movement.
4. Slowly lower your legs back down to the starting position. Keep your movements controlled and deliberate.
5. Repeat the exercise for 10-15 reps, or until you feel fatigued.

Here are some tips to keep in mind while performing hanging leg lifts with the Pilates bar:

- Focus on engaging your core muscles throughout the entire movement. Keep your abs tight and your back straight to prevent swinging or cheating.
- Don't use momentum to lift your legs. Instead, rely on your core strength to control the movement.
- If you have trouble keeping your legs straight, you can bend your knees slightly. However, make sure to keep your movements slow and controlled.

Plank with Row

It targets your core, back, arms, and shoulders, making it a full-body workout that requires strength, stability, and control.

To perform the plank with row:

1. Start in a high plank position with your hands holding onto the Pilates bar and your feet shoulder-width apart.

2. Engage your core and glutes, keeping your body in a straight line from head to heels.
3. Keep your elbows close to your body and slowly pull the Pilates bar towards your chest, squeezing your shoulder blades together.
4. Lower the Pilates bar back down to the starting position.
5. Repeat the row on the opposite side.
6. Continue alternating rows for the desired number of reps.

Tips:

- Keep your elbows close to your body to prevent any twisting in the torso.
- Make sure to engage your core throughout the exercise to maintain proper form and stability.
- Use a lighter resistance on the Pilates bar to start and gradually increase as you get stronger and more comfortable with the exercise.
- Focus on quality over quantity, making sure each rep is performed with control and proper form.

The Single Leg Circle

This workout targets the lower body, particularly the hip flexors, glutes, and inner thighs, it should only be performed by experienced Pilates practitioners who have mastered the basic Pilates bar workout exercises and have good hip and leg flexibility.

Here's how to perform the single leg circle:

1. Start by lying on your back with your legs straight and your arms at your sides. Place your hands on the Pilates bar above your head and engage your core.
2. Lift your right leg off the mat and extend it towards the ceiling. Keep your left leg on the mat and your left foot flexed.
3. Inhale and circle your right leg to the right, keeping it straight and reaching as far as you can without moving your pelvis. Exhale and circle your leg back to the starting position.
4. Repeat the circle in the opposite direction, circling your right leg to the left.
5. Complete 5-10 circles in each direction and then switch legs.

Here are some tips to keep in mind while performing the single leg circle:

- Keep your pelvis stable throughout the exercise. You should feel your core working to keep your lower back from arching off the mat.
- Focus on using your hip flexors and inner thighs to control the movement of your leg. Avoid using momentum or swinging your leg.
- Keep your shoulders relaxed and your neck long.
- Breathe deeply and consistently throughout the exercise, inhaling as you circle your leg to the side and exhaling as you circle back to the starting position.

Side Plank with Hip Lift

This exercise requires a high level of balance, core strength, and stability, so it is not recommended for beginners.

Here are the steps to perform a side plank with hip lift:

1. Start by placing your pilates bar on the floor and lie on your right side with your legs straight and stacked on top of each other. Place your right forearm on the ground perpendicular to your body, elbow directly below your shoulder. Your left hand can rest on your left hip.
2. Engage your core muscles, lift your hips off the ground, and come into a side plank position. Your body should form a straight line from your head to your heels.
3. Lower your hips towards the ground, but don't touch it. Then, lift your hips back up towards the ceiling, engaging your oblique muscles to perform a hip lift. Your body should remain in a straight line from head to heels.
4. Repeat the hip lift for 10-15 reps, then switch to the other side and repeat the exercise.

Here are some important things to keep in mind while performing the side plank with hip lift:

- Keep your shoulders down and away from your ears. Don't shrug them up towards your neck.
- Engage your core muscles throughout the exercise, and keep your body in a straight line from head to heels.
- Keep your neck in a neutral position, looking straight ahead.
- Breathe deeply and evenly throughout the exercise.
- If you're having trouble balancing, you can modify the exercise by placing your bottom knee on the ground and performing the hip lift.

CHAPTER 5: PILATES BAR WORKOUT FOR SPECIFIC GOALS

Pilates for Weight Loss: The Connection between Pilates Bar Workout and Weight Loss

Pilates is often associated with developing a strong, toned body and improving posture and flexibility. However, it is not commonly associated with weight loss. Nevertheless, Pilates can be an excellent way to lose weight, as it can help to burn calories, increase metabolism, and build lean muscle mass.

In this section, we will explore the connection between Pilates Bar Workout and weight loss, including the science behind how it works, the best Pilates Bar Workout exercises for weight loss, and tips for incorporating Pilates into your weight loss journey.

How Pilates Bar Workout Helps with Weight Loss:

Burn Calories: One of the primary ways Pilates Bar Workout can aid in weight loss is by helping to burn calories. Pilates Bar Workout is a form of exercise that can get your heart rate up and keep it elevated for an extended period. When you engage in any form of physical activity, your body burns calories, which can lead to weight loss over time.

Increase Metabolism: Pilates Bar Workout can also help to increase your metabolism. When you build lean muscle mass through Pilates Bar Workout, your body will burn more calories at rest. This means that even when you are not exercising, your body will be burning calories at a higher rate.

Build Lean Muscle Mass: Pilates Bar Workout is excellent for building lean muscle mass, which can contribute to weight loss. The more muscle you have, the more calories your body will burn, even when you are not exercising. Additionally, lean muscle mass takes up less space than fat, so you will look leaner and more toned even if you don't lose a lot of weight on the scale.

Best Pilates Bar Workout Exercises for Weight Loss

Plank Jacks

Plank Jacks are an effective Pilates Bar workout exercise that can help with weight loss by increasing cardiovascular endurance and burning calories. They target the core, arms, and legs while also engaging the cardiovascular system. Here's how to perform the Pilates Bar workout Plank Jacks:

Step 1: Start in a high plank position with your hands on the Pilates Bar and your feet hip-distance apart.

Step 2: Engage your core and keep your back straight as you jump both feet out to the sides, wider than hip-distance apart, while maintaining the high plank position.

Step 3: Quickly jump both feet back together to return to the starting position.

Step 4: Repeat this movement for 30 seconds to 1 minute, or as many reps as you can while maintaining good form.

Tips:

- Keep your core engaged and your back straight throughout the exercise to protect your lower back.
- Make sure your Pilates Bar is stable and secure to avoid any accidents or injuries.
- To make the exercise more challenging, you can add a push-up after each plank jack, or try performing the exercise on one leg at a time.

Jumping Jacks

Jumping jacks are a classic exercise that you might remember from your school days, but did you know that they can be a great addition to your Pilates bar workout for weight loss? Jumping jacks are a cardiovascular exercise that can help you burn calories and improve your overall fitness level.

How to Perform Pilates Bar Workout Jumping Jacks

1. Start by standing with your feet together and your Pilates bar held at your chest level with your hands.

2. Engage your core muscles and jump your feet out to the sides, while simultaneously lifting your Pilates bar overhead.
3. As you land, bring your feet back together and lower the Pilates bar back down to your chest.
4. Repeat this movement for a set amount of time or reps.

Tips for Performing Pilates Bar Workout Jumping Jacks

- Keep your core engaged throughout the exercise to maintain proper form and prevent injury.
- Land softly with your feet to avoid jarring your joints.
- Focus on your breathing, inhaling as you jump out and exhaling as you jump back in.
- If you have any knee or joint issues, you may want to avoid jumping jacks or modify the exercise by stepping out to the sides instead of jumping.

Lunge with Bicep Curls

This exercise combines strength training with cardio, making it a great calorie-burning workout.

To perform the Lunge with Bicep Curls, you will need a Pilates Bar and a set of light to medium dumbbells. Here are the steps to follow:

1. Stand with your feet hip-distance apart, holding the Pilates Bar in front of your thighs with an underhand grip.
2. Step your right foot forward and lower into a lunge, bending both knees to 90 degrees. Make sure your front knee is aligned over your ankle, and your back knee is hovering just above the ground.

3. As you lower into the lunge, simultaneously curl the dumbbells up to your shoulders, keeping your elbows close to your sides.
4. Pause for a moment at the bottom of the lunge, then press through your front heel to stand back up, lowering the dumbbells back down to your sides.
5. Repeat the lunge with your left leg forward, curling the dumbbells up as you lower down and lowering them back down as you stand up.
6. Alternate lunging with your right and left legs for 10-12 reps on each side, for a total of 20-24 lunges.

When performing this exercise, keep your core engaged and your chest lifted. Focus on keeping your weight in your front heel as you press back up to standing. You can also increase the intensity of this exercise by using heavier weights or increasing the speed of your lunges.

Pilates Sit-ups

This exercise is also known as the roll-up exercise and is an advanced Pilates move that requires proper form and technique to prevent injury.

Here Is a step-by-step guide on how to perform Pilates sit-ups using the Pilates Bar:

1. Start by lying on your back on a Pilates mat or a soft surface with your legs straight and together. Extend your arms above your head, holding the Pilates Bar with both hands, shoulder-width apart.

2. Inhale deeply and engage your core muscles by pulling your belly button towards your spine.
3. Exhale and slowly lift your head, neck, and shoulders off the mat, rolling up one vertebra at a time. At the same time, lift the Pilates Bar towards the ceiling and keep your arms straight.
4. Pause at the top of the movement, hold for a second, and then inhale as you slowly lower your torso and the Pilates Bar back down to the mat.
5. Repeat the movement for 8-10 reps.

Tips and considerations:

- Make sure to keep your feet flat on the mat and avoid lifting them off the ground during the movement.
- Keep your shoulders relaxed and away from your ears throughout the exercise.
- Focus on using your abdominal muscles to roll up and down, not your neck or shoulders.
- Keep the Pilates Bar stable and avoid swinging it during the movement.

The Standing Oblique Crunch

This exercise helps to tone the waistline, improve posture, and increase overall core strength. It can also be an effective way to burn calories and aid in weight loss efforts.

To perform the standing oblique crunch, follow these steps:

1. Stand with your feet hip-width apart, holding the Pilates Bar with both hands, arms extended overhead.
2. Engage your core muscles and keep your shoulders down and back throughout the exercise.
3. Slowly lower the Pilates Bar to one side of your body, bending at the waist and keeping your hips stable.
4. As you lower the Pilates Bar, lift the opposite knee towards the elbow on the same side of the body. Your knee and elbow should meet in the middle, engaging your oblique muscles.
5. Hold for a moment before returning to the starting position.
6. Repeat on the other side, alternating sides for each repetition.

Avoid leaning too far to one side or arching your back, as this can strain your lower back muscles. Keep your movements slow and controlled, and only lower the Pilates Bar as far as you can while maintaining proper form.

The Burpee with Pilates Bar Row

To perform this exercise, follow these steps:

1. Start by holding the Pilates bar with an overhand grip. Stand with your feet shoulder-width apart and your knees slightly bent.
2. Lower the bar to the floor, bending at the hips and knees until you reach a squatting position with the bar touching the floor.
3. From this position, kick your legs back into a push-up position, keeping your arms straight.

4. Perform a push-up, keeping your elbows close to your body.
5. After the push-up, jump your legs back towards your hands and stand up, lifting the bar with you as you do.
6. As you stand up, lift the bar to chest height and perform a row, pulling the bar towards your chest and squeezing your shoulder blades together.
7. Lower the bar to the starting position and repeat the exercise.

Tips for Proper Form:

- Keep your back straight and your abs engaged throughout the exercise.
- Keep your elbows close to your body during the push-up and row.
- When standing up from the push-up position, use your legs to help you, not just your arms.
- Focus on squeezing your shoulder blades together during the row to fully engage your back muscles.

This exercise is an excellent addition to any weight loss program, as it not only burns calories, but also helps build muscle, which in turn helps increase your metabolism. Incorporate this exercise into your Pilates bar workout routine and watch as the pounds melt away.

Remember, weight loss is not just about exercise, but also about making healthy lifestyle choices such as eating a balanced diet and staying hydrated.

Pilates for Athletes: Incorporating Pilates Bar Workout into Your Athletic Training

Whether you are a runner, basketball player, soccer player, or any other athlete, incorporating Pilates Bar exercises into your training can help you take your performance to the next level. Here's everything you need to know about Pilates Bar workouts for athletes.

The Benefits of Pilates Bar Workouts for Athletes

Improved Core Strength: Many Pilates Bar exercises focus on strengthening the core muscles. A strong core is essential for athletes, as it helps stabilize the body and transfer power from the lower body to the upper body.

Better Balance and Stability: Pilates Bar exercises also improve balance and stability, which are important for all athletes. Better balance and stability can help prevent falls and injuries, and improve overall performance.

Increased Flexibility: Flexibility is crucial for athletes, as it allows them to move more freely and avoid injuries. Pilates Bar workouts incorporate a range of stretches and movements that can help improve flexibility.

Reduced Risk of Injury: Pilates Bar exercises focus on proper form and alignment, which can help athletes avoid injuries. By strengthening the muscles and improving balance, athletes can reduce their risk of injuries while performing their sport.

Improved Mental Focus: Pilates Bar workouts require mental focus and concentration, which can help athletes improve their focus and concentration during their sport.

Plank with Arm and Leg Lift

Plank with Arm and Leg Lift is a challenging Pilates Bar workout that can help athletes improve their core strength, balance, and stability. Here's how to perform this exercise:

1. Start in a plank position with your hands on the Pilates Bar and your feet hip-distance apart. Keep your shoulders directly over your wrists and engage your core muscles.
2. Extend your right arm forward and your left leg backward, keeping them straight and parallel to the ground. Keep your hips level and your gaze down between your hands.
3. Hold this position for a few seconds, then return to the starting plank position.
4. Repeat with the left arm and right leg.
5. Continue alternating sides for several repetitions.

When performing Plank with Arm and Leg Lift, make sure to keep your hips level and your shoulders stable, without allowing your torso to twist or sag. Avoid holding your breath and focus on breathing deeply and evenly throughout the exercise.

Hip Bridge with Chest Press

This help athletes build strength in the glutes, hamstrings, and chest muscles. It also helps to improve core stability and balance.

To perform the exercise:

1. Lie on your back on a mat with your knees bent and your feet flat on the ground. Hold the Pilates bar with both hands and place it on your hips.
2. Inhale and press your hips up towards the ceiling, lifting your buttocks off the ground. Keep your feet and shoulders on the ground.
3. Exhale and slowly lower your hips back down to the ground, keeping your back straight and your core engaged.
4. Next, inhale and press the Pilates bar up towards the ceiling, extending your arms straight above your chest.
5. Exhale and slowly lower the Pilates bar back down towards your chest.
6. Repeat the hip bridge and chest press for 10-12 repetitions, or as many as you can while maintaining proper form.

Important things to keep in mind:

- Make sure your feet are hip-width apart and your knees are aligned with your ankles.
- Keep your shoulders relaxed and your chin tucked in towards your chest.
- Engage your core muscles throughout the exercise to help stabilize your body.
- Do not arch your back or lift your shoulders off the ground when pressing the Pilates bar.

- To make the exercise more challenging, you can increase the weight of the Pilates bar or add a resistance band around your thighs.

Forward Lunge with Rotation

Here's how to perform the exercise:

1. Start by standing tall with your feet hip-width apart and your Pilates bar held at chest height with your hands shoulder-width apart.
2. Take a big step forward with your right foot, lowering your body down into a lunge position. Make sure your front knee is directly above your ankle and your back knee is hovering just above the ground.
3. As you lower into the lunge, rotate your torso to the right, bringing the Pilates bar towards your right hip.
4. Pause for a moment, then return to the starting position by pushing through your right foot and straightening your leg. At the same time, rotate your torso back to center and bring the Pilates bar back to your chest.
5. Repeat on the other side, stepping forward with your left foot and rotating your torso to the left.

Tips:

- Keep your core engaged and your spine straight throughout the exercise.
- Focus on maintaining your balance as you rotate your torso.
- Make sure your knee stays aligned with your ankle to prevent injury.

- Exhale as you lunge forward and inhale as you return to the starting position.

Side Plank with Hip Dips

This exercise targets the obliques, hips, and shoulders, making it an effective full-body workout.

To perform this exercise, follow these steps:

1. Start by lying on your side with your legs straight and stacked on top of each other. Your elbow should be bent, and your forearm should be resting on the Pilates bar. Your other hand should be on your hip.
2. Engage your core and lift your hips off the ground, creating a straight line from your head to your feet. Your elbow should be directly under your shoulder.
3. Once you have found your balance, slowly dip your hips towards the ground, then raise them back up to the starting position. This movement is one hip dip.
4. Repeat the hip dips for 10 to 12 reps on one side, then switch to the other side and repeat.

Some things to keep in mind while performing this exercise:

- Keep your core engaged throughout the movement to maintain your balance.
- Make sure your elbow is directly under your shoulder to avoid putting unnecessary strain on your shoulder joint.

- If you find the exercise too challenging, you can modify it by bending your bottom leg and resting your knee on the ground.
- As you become more comfortable with the exercise, you can increase the number of hip dips or hold the side plank position for longer periods.

Reverse Lunge with Bicep Curl

To perform, follow these steps

1. Start by standing upright with your feet hip-width apart and your Pilates Bar resting comfortably on your shoulders, hands gripping the bar just outside your shoulders.
2. Take a step back with your right foot, bending both knees until your left knee forms a 90-degree angle and your right knee is hovering just above the ground.
3. As you lower into the lunge, simultaneously curl the Pilates Bar up towards your shoulders, engaging your biceps.
4. Pause for a moment at the bottom of the lunge, maintaining your balance and keeping your core tight.
5. Push through your left foot to rise back up to the starting position, lowering the Pilates Bar back down to your shoulders.
6. Repeat the exercise on the other side, taking a step back with your left foot and curling the Pilates Bar up towards your shoulders as you lower into the lunge.

Tips:

- Keep your chest lifted and your shoulders relaxed throughout the exercise.
- Keep your front knee stacked over your ankle, ensuring that it does not extend past your toes.
- Engage your core muscles to maintain your balance throughout the movement.
- Exhale as you lower into the lunge and curl the Pilates Bar up, inhale as you rise back up to the starting position.
- Start with a light Pilates Bar weight and increase as you become comfortable with the movement.

Single-Leg Deadlift

Single-Leg Deadlift is a great exercise for athletes as it strengthens the glutes, hamstrings, and lower back muscles, which are crucial for many sports movements such as sprinting, jumping, and changing direction. It also helps to improve balance and stability, making it an effective exercise for injury prevention.

Here's how to perform the Pilates Bar Single-Leg Deadlift:

1. Begin by standing tall with your feet hip-width apart and the Pilates bar resting on your shoulders behind your neck. Your hands should be holding the bar at each end, with your palms facing forward.
2. Shift your weight onto your left foot and lift your right foot off the ground, keeping your knee slightly bent.
3. Hinge forward from your hips, keeping your back straight and your core engaged. As you hinge forward, lift your right leg behind you until it is parallel to the ground.
4. Lower the Pilates bar towards the ground as you hinge forward, keeping it close to your body. Your arms should be

straight and your elbows should be pointing towards the ground.

5. Pause when you reach the bottom of the movement, then slowly return to the starting position, keeping your core engaged and your back straight.
6. Repeat for the desired number of repetitions, then switch sides and repeat with your left leg.

Tips:

- Start with a lighter weight Pilates bar and gradually increase the weight as you get stronger and more comfortable with the exercise.
- Keep your core engaged throughout the exercise to maintain balance and stability.
- Focus on keeping your back straight and hinging from your hips, rather than rounding your back.
- If you find it difficult to balance, try placing your free hand on a wall or chair for support.

Pilates for Stress Relief: The Role of Pilates Bar Workout in Reducing Stress and Anxiety

In today's fast-paced world, stress and anxiety are common among many individuals. While there are various ways to reduce stress and anxiety, one effective method is through exercise. Pilates Bar workouts can help in reducing stress and anxiety by calming the mind and improving overall well-being. In this section, we will explore the role of Pilates Bar workout in reducing stress and anxiety and discuss some effective exercises.

Research has shown that regular Pilates Bar workouts can reduce cortisol levels, a hormone associated with stress, and anxiety. This reduction in cortisol levels can help individuals feel more relaxed and reduce the physical symptoms of stress, such as muscle tension and headaches.

Effective Pilates Bar Workout Exercises for Stress Relief:

Roll Up

The Pilates Bar Roll Up is a great exercise for reducing stress and anxiety by promoting relaxation and mindfulness. Here's how to perform it:

1. Start by lying flat on your back on a mat with your legs straight and your arms extended above your head, holding the Pilates bar with both hands.
2. Inhale and engage your core muscles, then slowly roll up one vertebra at a time, keeping your arms extended in front of you and your feet on the mat.
3. Exhale as you reach forward towards your toes, keeping your spine straight and your neck relaxed.
4. Inhale and slowly roll back down one vertebra at a time until you're back in the starting position with your arms extended above your head.
5. Repeat this movement for several reps, focusing on your breath and maintaining a slow, controlled pace.

Here are some tips to keep in mind while performing the Pilates Bar Roll Up:

- Make sure to keep your core engaged throughout the movement, as this will help you maintain control and stability.
- Keep your neck relaxed and your gaze focused towards your toes as you roll up, rather than straining your neck to look forward.
- If you're having trouble rolling up smoothly, you can bend your knees slightly or use a Pilates ball or cushion to support your lower back.
- As you become more comfortable with the movement, you can increase the challenge by holding the roll-up position for a few seconds before rolling back down.

Leg Circles

Pilates Bar Leg circles is a great exercise to reduce stress and anxiety while toning your legs and improving flexibility. This exercise targets the glutes, inner and outer thighs, and hip flexors. Here is how to perform it:

1. Start by lying on your back with your legs extended and your Pilates Bar resting on the tops of your feet. Your arms should be extended out to your sides, palms facing down.
2. Engage your core and lift your legs up towards the ceiling, creating a 90-degree angle at the hips and knees.
3. Slowly begin to draw small circles with your legs, making sure to keep your movements controlled and fluid. As you circle

your legs, maintain the 90-degree angle at your hips and knees.
4. After 10-15 circles in one direction, switch directions and complete another 10-15 circles.
5. Once you have completed both directions, lower your legs back down to the starting position.

Tips:

- Focus on engaging your core throughout the exercise to help stabilize your body and maintain control.
- Keep your movements small and controlled, and avoid any jerky or sudden movements.
- If you feel any discomfort in your lower back, try placing a small pillow or cushion under your tailbone for support.

You can make this exercise more challenging by adding ankle weights or increasing the number of circles you complete in each direction.

Spine Stretch Forward

The Pilates Bar Spine Stretch Forward is an excellent exercise for relieving stress and tension in the body. It targets the spine, shoulders, and neck, which are common areas where stress accumulates. Here's how to perform this exercise:

1. Sit upright on a mat with your legs extended in front of you and your feet flexed. Place the Pilates bar in front of you, resting it on the ground.
2. Hold the Pilates bar with both hands, with your palms facing down and your hands shoulder-width apart.

3. Inhale and lengthen your spine, reaching the top of your head towards the ceiling.
4. Exhale and begin to roll your spine forward, starting with your head and neck. Keep your arms straight and your shoulders relaxed.
5. Continue to roll forward, bringing your torso towards your legs, until you reach a comfortable stretch. You should feel a stretch in your spine and the backs of your legs.
6. Hold this position for a few breaths, then inhale and slowly roll back up to the starting position.
7. Repeat this exercise for several repetitions, focusing on your breath and the release of tension in your body.

Some tips to keep in mind when performing this exercise:

- Keep your shoulders relaxed and away from your ears.
- Avoid rounding your spine too much, as this can cause strain.
- If you have any neck or back injuries, speak with a healthcare professional before attempting this exercise.
- Focus on breathing deeply and slowly to help calm your mind and release tension in your body.

Swimming

Here's how to perform it:

1. Start by lying face down on the mat with your legs extended and arms holding the Pilates bar above your head.
2. Engage your core and lift your arms and legs slightly off the mat.

3. Begin to flutter your arms and legs up and down in a controlled motion, as if you were swimming.
4. As you flutter, keep your gaze down towards the mat and ensure that your neck is in a neutral position.
5. Breathe in deeply and exhale as you flutter your arms and legs.
6. Repeat this motion for 10-12 repetitions or as long as you can hold it.
7. Lower your arms and legs to the mat and rest.

Swan

Swan is an excellent exercise for reducing stress and tension in the upper body. It targets the muscles of the back, shoulders, and arms while promoting relaxation and deep breathing.

To perform the Pilates Bar Swan:

1. Begin by lying face down on a mat with your legs extended and feet hip-width apart. Hold the Pilates bar with an overhand grip, with your hands shoulder-width apart and arms extended in front of you.
2. Inhale as you engage your core and lift your chest and arms off the mat, keeping your gaze forward and neck long.
3. Exhale as you lower your chest and arms back down to the mat, keeping your shoulders relaxed.
4. Repeat for a set of 8-10 reps.

Tips to keep in mind:

- Focus on lifting your chest and arms with your back muscles, rather than using your arms to pull yourself up.

- Keep your shoulders relaxed and away from your ears throughout the movement.
- Breathe deeply and smoothly, inhaling as you lift and exhaling as you lower.

Chest Expansion

Here's how to perform it:

1. Begin by standing with your feet hip-width apart and your Pilates bar at chest height in front of you.
2. Hold the bar with both hands, keeping your arms straight and your palms facing down.
3. Inhale and pull the Pilates bar towards your chest, keeping your shoulders relaxed and down.
4. Exhale and slowly push the Pilates bar away from your chest, stretching your arms straight out in front of you.
5. Inhale and repeat the movement, pulling the bar towards your chest and exhaling as you push it away.

Here are some things to keep in mind while performing the Pilates bar chest expansion:

- Focus on keeping your shoulders relaxed and down throughout the movement.
- Keep your arms straight and engage your core muscles to maintain proper form.
- Breathe deeply and evenly throughout the exercise.
- If you have any shoulder or neck injuries, be sure to consult with a healthcare professional before attempting this exercise.

Seated Forward Fold

The Pilates bar seated forward fold is a great exercise for reducing stress and anxiety. It stretches the entire back of your body, including your hamstrings, glutes, and spine, which helps to release tension and promote relaxation. Here's how to perform it:

1. Begin seated on the floor with your legs extended straight out in front of you and the Pilates bar in your hands.
2. Inhale, sit up tall, and reach the Pilates bar out in front of you.
3. Exhale and slowly fold forward, keeping your spine long and your shoulders relaxed.
4. As you fold forward, slide the Pilates bar down your legs, keeping your hands and arms relaxed.
5. Continue to fold forward until you feel a comfortable stretch in the backs of your legs and spine. Hold for several breaths.
6. To come out of the pose, inhale and slowly roll up through your spine, keeping your head and neck relaxed.

Here are some tips to keep in mind while performing the Pilates bar seated forward fold:

- If you have tight hamstrings, you may not be able to fold forward very far. That's okay! Only go as far as feels comfortable for your body.
- Avoid rounding your spine as you fold forward. Keep your spine long and your shoulders relaxed.
- Don't force the stretch. You should feel a comfortable stretch, but if you feel any pain, come out of the pose immediately.

- Use your breath to help deepen the stretch. Inhale to lengthen your spine, and exhale to fold forward.

CHAPTER 7: RECOVERY AND COOL-DOWN

The Importance of Recovery

In the world of fitness, recovery is often an overlooked component of a well-rounded workout routine. Many people focus solely on the intensity and duration of their workouts, neglecting the crucial role that recovery plays in achieving optimal health and fitness. In fact, recovery is just as important as exercise itself, and neglecting recovery can lead to injury, burnout, and suboptimal results.

As much as we enjoy pushing ourselves during a workout, it's important to remember that recovery is just as important as exercise. Recovery is the period of time between workouts when your body is repairing and rebuilding itself. This is the time when your muscles recover from the stress they endured during your workout and when your body adapts to the exercise you just performed.

So, what exactly is recovery? Recovery refers to the process of allowing your body to rest and repair after physical activity. During exercise, your body experiences micro-tears in your muscles, which then require time to heal and become stronger. Additionally, your body's energy stores are depleted during exercise, and recovery allows your body to replenish those stores.

There are many different strategies for recovery, including rest, hydration, nutrition, and active recovery techniques such as foam rolling, stretching, and massage. Let's take a closer look at each of these strategies and their importance in the recovery process.

Rest: Rest is perhaps the most critical component of recovery. Your body needs time to heal and repair itself after physical activity, and without adequate rest, you increase your risk of injury, illness, and burnout. This means getting enough sleep each night, taking rest days between workouts, and listening to your body when it tells you it needs a break.

Hydration: Hydration is also crucial for recovery. When you exercise, you sweat, and you lose fluids and electrolytes. Replenishing those fluids and electrolytes is essential for maintaining proper bodily functions and helping your body recover. Aim to drink at least 8-10 glasses of water per day, and consider adding electrolyte-rich beverages such as coconut water or sports drinks to your hydration routine.

Nutrition: Proper nutrition is another critical component of recovery. After exercise, your body needs protein and carbohydrates to replenish energy stores and repair muscle tissue. Aim to consume a balanced meal or snack containing both protein and carbohydrates within 30 minutes to an hour after your workout. Additionally, be sure to consume plenty of fruits and vegetables, which provide essential vitamins and minerals that aid in recovery.

Active Recovery Techniques: In addition to rest, hydration, and nutrition, active recovery techniques such as foam rolling, stretching, and massage can also help aid in recovery. Foam rolling can help break up tight spots in your muscles, while stretching can help increase flexibility and range of motion. Massage can also help reduce muscle soreness and tension.

It's important to note that recovery is not a one-size-fits-all process. The amount of recovery you need will vary based on your individual fitness level, workout intensity, and overall health. Listen to your body and adjust your recovery routine accordingly.

A Relaxing Cool-Down Sequence for Pilates Bar Workout

As I have said, cooling down after a workout is just as important as warming up, but often overlooked. Pilates Bar workout is no exception, and a proper cool-down sequence can help reduce muscle soreness, prevent injury, and promote relaxation. In this section, we will explore a relaxing cool-down sequence for Pilates Bar workout that will leave you feeling refreshed and rejuvenated.

Seated Forward Fold with Side Stretch

Seated forward fold with side stretch is a gentle and calming cool-down exercise that helps to release tension and increase flexibility in the hips, hamstrings, and lower back. Here's how to perform it:

1. Begin by sitting on your mat with your legs extended in front of you and your Pilates bar resting across your thighs. Sit up tall and engage your core muscles.
2. As you inhale, lift your arms overhead, lengthening your spine and reaching your fingertips towards the ceiling.
3. As you exhale, hinge forward from your hips, keeping your spine long and your core engaged. Allow your hands to rest on your shins, ankles, or the floor in front of you, depending on your flexibility.
4. Hold this forward fold for a few breaths, then slowly walk your hands to the right side of your body, keeping your left hip anchored to the mat. Hold for a few breaths, feeling a stretch along the left side of your body.
5. Inhale as you come back to center, then exhale and walk your hands to the left side of your body, feeling a stretch along the right side of your body.
6. Slowly come back to center and release your hands from your Pilates bar. Roll up to a seated position, and take a few deep breaths to center yourself.

Here are some key things to keep in mind as you perform seated forward fold with side stretch:

- This is a gentle stretch, so take your time and move slowly.
- If you have tight hamstrings or lower back pain, you may need to keep a slight bend in your knees as you fold forward.
- You can use your Pilates bar to help support you in the forward fold, but don't force yourself deeper than feels comfortableAs you walk your hands to the side, keep your sit bones anchored to the mat to maintain stability and prevent tipping to one side.

- Remember to breathe deeply and stay present in the moment as you release tension and calm your mind.

Downward-facing Dog

Downward-facing dog is a popular yoga pose that is also commonly incorporated into Pilates Bar workouts as a relaxing cool-down exercise. Here's how to perform this pose:

1. Start on all fours, with your hands shoulder-width apart and your knees hip-width apart. Your fingers should be spread wide with your middle fingers pointing straight ahead.
2. As you exhale, lift your hips up and back, straightening your arms and legs as much as you can. Your body should resemble an inverted V-shape.
3. Engage your core and press your heels down towards the mat, feeling a stretch through the back of your legs.
4. Keep your head and neck relaxed, and try to lengthen your spine as much as possible.
5. Hold the pose for several deep breaths, then release and come back to all fours.

Here are some tips to keep in mind:

- If you have tight hamstrings or lower back pain, you can bend your knees slightly to help release the tension.
- If your wrists bother you, you can modify the pose by coming onto your forearms instead of your hands.
- You can also experiment with widening or narrowing your stance to find what feels most comfortable for you.

The Supine Twist

The Supine Twist is a gentle and relaxing cool-down exercise that helps to release tension in the spine and hips. Here's how to perform it:

1. Lie down on your back with your legs extended and your arms out to the sides, palms facing down.
2. Bring your right knee in towards your chest and hold onto it with your left hand.
3. Use your right hand to gently guide your right knee across your body towards the left side, keeping your shoulder blades on the mat.
4. Hold the stretch for 5-10 deep breaths, feeling the stretch in your lower back and outer hip.
5. Slowly release and repeat on the other side, bringing your left knee in towards your chest and using your right hand to guide it across your body towards the right side.
6. Repeat on each side for 2-3 rounds.

Things to keep in mind:

- If you have any pre-existing spinal or hip injuries, please consult with your healthcare provider before attempting this exercise.
- Don't force the stretch – it should feel gentle and comfortable.
- Keep both shoulders on the mat throughout the exercise.
- Focus on deep breathing and allow yourself to fully relax into the stretch.

Happy Baby Pose

Happy Baby Pose is a relaxing yoga pose that can be incorporated into your Pilates Bar workout cool-down sequence to help release tension in the hips and lower back. Here's how to perform the pose:

1. Lie down on your back with your knees bent and your feet flat on the floor.
2. Take a deep breath in and as you exhale, draw your knees in towards your chest.
3. Reach your arms inside your legs and grab hold of the outside edges of your feet.
4. Keeping your feet flexed, gently pull your knees down towards your armpits. Your shins should be perpendicular to the ground.
5. Lengthen your spine by pressing your tailbone down towards the ground.
6. Relax your shoulders and let them rest on the mat.
7. Hold the pose for 30-60 seconds, breathing deeply.
8. To release, gently let go of your feet and extend your legs out onto the mat.

Things to keep in mind:

- If you have tight hips or lower back pain, you may find it difficult to hold onto your feet. In this case, you can place your hands on your shins or use a strap to hold onto your feet.
- If your neck feels strained, you can rest your head on a small pillow or folded blanket.
- Be sure to breathe deeply and focus on relaxing your body as you hold the pose.

Savasana

Savasana, also known as Corpse Pose, is a relaxing cool-down pose that allows your body to relax and release any tension that may have built up during your workout, while also allowing you to quiet your mind and enter a state of deep relaxation.

To perform Savasana, start by lying on your back with your arms at your sides and your palms facing up. Your legs should be straight, and your feet should be hip-distance apart. Allow your body to sink into the ground, and close your eyes.

Take a few deep breaths, inhaling through your nose and exhaling through your mouth. As you exhale, allow your body to release any tension or stress that you may be holding onto.

Once you have settled into the pose, focus on relaxing each part of your body, starting at your toes and working your way up to the top of your head. Allow each muscle to release any tension that it may be holding onto.

Stay in this pose for as long as you like, but aim for at least five to ten minutes. When you are ready to come out of the pose, slowly bring your awareness back to your body, wiggle your fingers and toes, and gently roll onto your right side. Take a few deep breaths before slowly sitting up.

Hip Flexor Stretch

Hip flexors are a group of muscles that connect your upper body to your legs, and they are responsible for movements such as walking, running, and bending. When these muscles become tight, they can cause pain in the lower back, hips, and knees.

To perform the Hip Flexor Stretch, follow these steps:

1. Start in a lunge position with your right foot forward and your left leg extended behind you. Keep your back straight and your hips facing forward.
2. Engage your core and shift your weight forward onto your right leg. You should feel a stretch in your left hip flexor.
3. To deepen the stretch, reach your arms up overhead and lean back slightly. Hold for 30 seconds.
4. Release the stretch by bringing your hands back down to the floor on either side of your right foot.
5. Repeat on the other side by switching the position of your legs.

Remember to keep your back straight, engage your core, and avoid arching your back. If you feel any pain or discomfort, ease off the stretch and seek advice from a certified Pilates instructor.

PILATES BAR WORKOUT FOR LIFE: CONTINUING YOUR PILATES JOURNEY

Congratulations on completing your Pilates Bar workout program! You have accomplished so much in your journey towards improved fitness, strength, flexibility, and overall well-being. But your journey doesn't end here. It's time to transition into the next phase of your Pilates journey: incorporating Pilates Bar workouts into your daily life.

In this section, we'll discuss how you can continue to make Pilates a part of your life beyond just completing a program. We'll explore different ways you can practice Pilates at home or at the gym, how to stay motivated, and how to continue progressing and challenging yourself.

Set Realistic Goals

The first step in continuing your Pilates journey is setting realistic goals for yourself. This means taking into account your current fitness level, any injuries or limitations you may have, and your lifestyle. Set goals that are achievable and sustainable for you, and don't compare yourself to others. Your Pilates journey is unique to you, and that's something to be proud of.

Mix It Up

To keep things interesting and avoid boredom, mix up your Pilates Bar workouts by incorporating different exercises, props, and Pilates styles. This not only helps prevent plateaus in your progress but also allows you to challenge your body in new ways. Consider trying out a reformer Pilates class or adding resistance bands to your routine.

Find a Pilates Buddy

Working out with a friend can make your Pilates Bar workouts more fun and motivating. You can hold each other accountable and encourage each other to keep pushing forward. If you can't find a workout buddy, consider joining a Pilates community online or in-person to connect with like-minded individuals and share your progress.

Listen to Your Body

It's important to listen to your body and take rest days when needed. Overexerting yourself can lead to injury and burnout. Incorporating gentle Pilates stretches or foam rolling into your routine can also help with muscle soreness and promote relaxation.

Make It a Habit

Consistency is key to seeing continued progress in your Pilates Bar workout journey. Make Pilates a habit by scheduling it into your weekly routine and treating it as a non-negotiable appointment with yourself. Whether it's early in the morning or after work, find a time that works best for you and stick to it.

Invest in Quality Equipment

Investing in quality Pilates equipment, such as a Pilates Bar or reformer, can take your practice to the next level. Having your own equipment at home allows you to practice Pilates on your own time and at your own pace. Consider consulting with a Pilates instructor or trainer to find the best equipment for your needs.

Continue Learning

Pilates Bar workouts have endless possibilities for progression and growth. Continue learning and expanding your knowledge by taking workshops, classes, or online courses. This not only helps prevent boredom but also allows you to deepen your understanding of Pilates and how it can benefit your body and mind.

Made in United States
Troutdale, OR
05/01/2024

19578372R10080